HOPE

September 2018

I0829855

After Brain Injury

HOPE
MAGAZINE

"Supporting the Brain Injury Community"

Welcome

HOPE MAGAZINE

Serving the Brain Injury Community

September 2018

Publisher
David A. Grant

Editor
Sarah Grant

Contributing Writers

Michelle Bartlett
Sarah Grant
Ric Johnson
Katherine A. Kimes
Cynthia Lim
Norma Myers
Coral-Lynn Rubino
Ellen Shaughnessy
Lisa Yee

FREE subscriptions at
www.HopeAfterBrainInjury.com

Welcome to the September 2018 issue of HOPE Magazine!

When brain injury strikes, there are many who are affected. From spouses to children, to employers and family members, all feel the effects in some way, making brain injury unlike most medical conditions.

One of the primary objectives of HOPE Magazine is to offer real insight about brain injury by those who best understand it. This month's issue features stories by several brain injury survivors, offering unparalleled insight into the day-to-day challenges faced by millions.

We are also pleased to share caregiver and family member stories including one by my wife Sarah aptly titled *Have You See the Bread*? In her story, she shares a snapshot of what it's like to live with a brain injury survivor – me!

Even after all these years, I was taken aback seeing things through her eyes!

I hope you come away from this issue with renewed hope.

Peace,

David A. Grant
Publisher

Contents

"Success is walking from failure to failure with no loss of enthusiasm."

~Winston Churchill

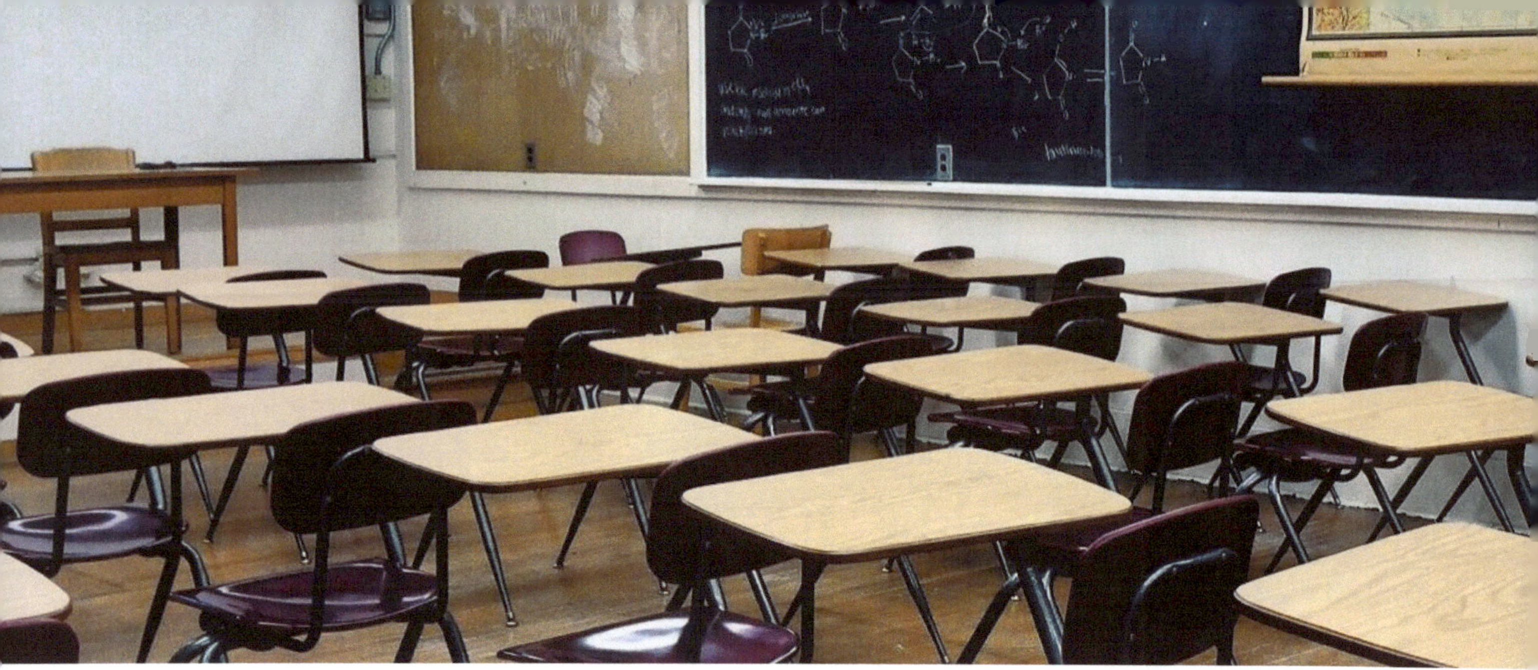

Learning Something New

By Ellen Shaughnessy

"It is never too late to learn something new," my dad said to me often. He was always open to new thoughts, new experiences, and new people. Never did I think that I would learn the meaning of that saying so forcefully.

Before my TBI, I was a nursing supervisor in charge of a large acute care medical facility. My responsibilities were all-encompassing and required that I make multiple decisions every hour of a twelve-hour shift. I needed to constantly change priorities, readjust my plans and formulate new ones.

Taking charge and being in control was part of my personality. All that changed on October 27, 2015. My TBI occurred due to an assault by a patient and ended a very satisfying and fulfilling forty-two-year nursing career. In the blink of an eye, my world turned upside down. It changed from taking charge of everything to not recalling when or if I had showered, conversations from ten minutes before, whether I took my meds, or even events from my life.

> Driving, shopping, reading, finding my words and staying awake became almost impossible and verv difficult.

Driving, shopping, reading, finding my words and staying awake became almost impossible and very difficult. For a long time, I didn't recognize that any of this was occurring and thought I was "fine!"

Needless to say, I was NOT easy to live with as I thought my perceptions of events in my life were correct. Asking for and accepting help was very difficult as I thought that I could figure things out and deal with my issues myself.

After cognitive therapy, physical therapy (for balance, dizziness and neck pain), and much research on my own, I had a more realistic understanding of my issues. I needed help on this roller coaster journey. That help came in a very unexpected way.

After eighteen months, I decided to attend a TBI support group meeting. The meeting had been offered to me many times, but I didn't feel groups were for me as I was "fine."

The meeting blew me away! There were other people who had my same issues. Not only were they able to laugh at themselves, but they understood immediately the issues others talked about. You were instantly accepted just because you showed up. Members of the group were at various stages of their recovery. It was so helpful to me to recognize not only where I had been but also where I could get to with patience, time and the support of these wonderful people.

I had been struggling a lot with my sense of purpose as I could no longer work. That was devastating to me. A few of the others were also feeling this way. It was comforting to me to not feel alone in this and to have someone to talk with about it who understood my upset. It gave me a new perspective on my symptoms, hope that I could improve and humbled me to be a witness to their courage.

Now, I look forward to the monthly meetings and try my best not to miss one. It is a constant surprise what I might learn and who I might meet. The most surprising and delightful occurrence has been that I have made friendships that are more meaningful to me than some I have had for a long time.

These fellow TBI survivors have exhibited a resourcefulness, zest for life and some very interesting ways to manage their lives.

The experience is different every month and never ceases to amaze me with the comfort and mindfulness that I come away with each time. Many of us are blessed to have great support people but there is such comfort in not needing to explain how you feel because my support group just gets it.

There have been many lessons that I have learned on this journey in the three years since my new life started. Some have been hard, hurtful, humbling and very upsetting but I can say that one of the joys has been finding my group. As my dad shared over the years, it was a wonderful lesson to find that it is never too late to learn something new. Thanks Dad.

Meet Ellen Shaughnessy

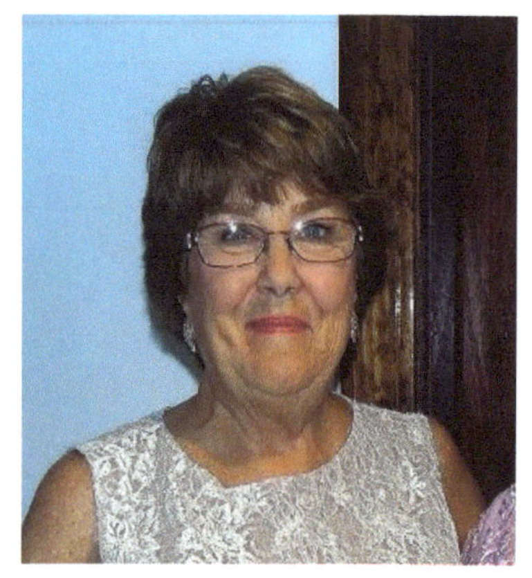

Ellen resides in Massachusetts and is a wife, mother and grandmother. Due to an assault at work in October 2015, she is now a retired RN. Friends, family, traveling, crafts and reading now occupy her time, as well as list making and putting everything in her calendar to jog her memory. She has previously written an article published in "Surviving Brain Injury."

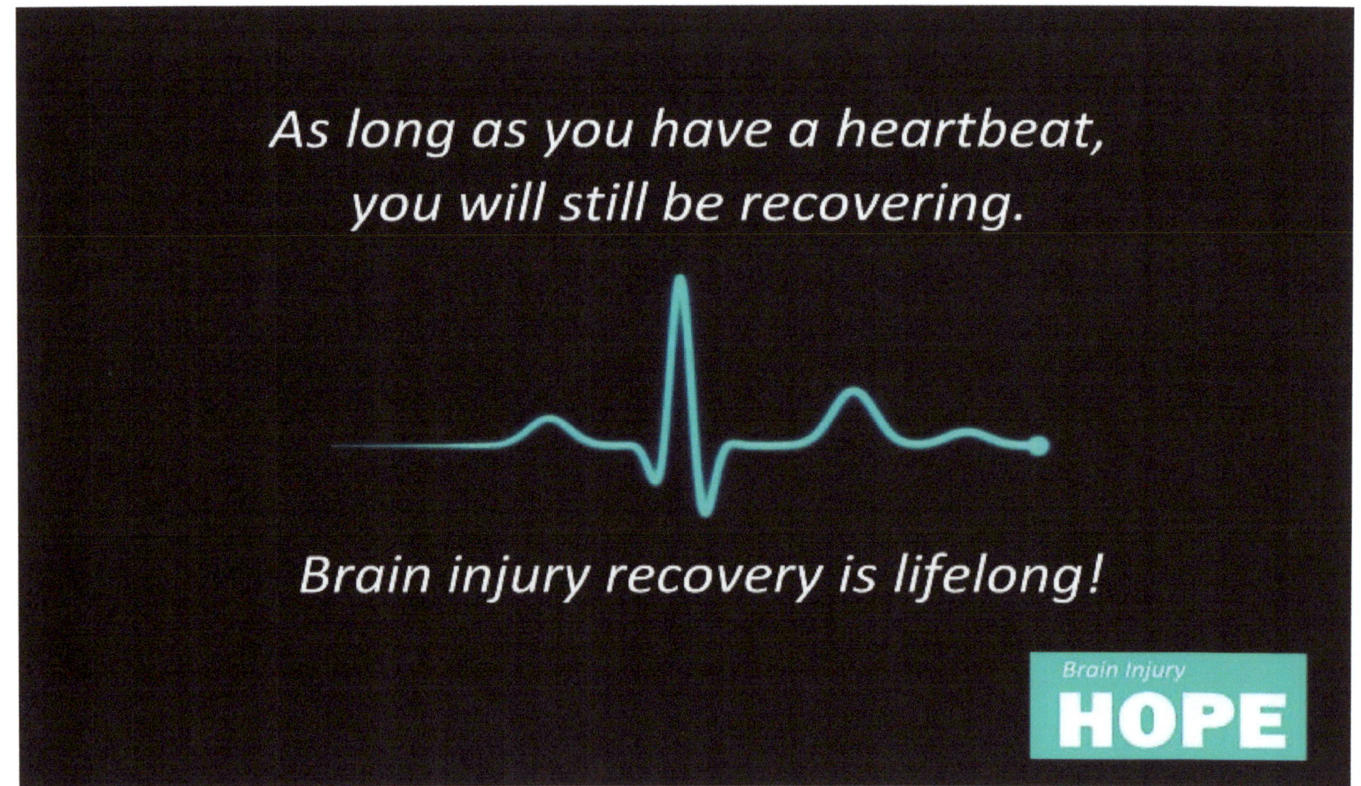

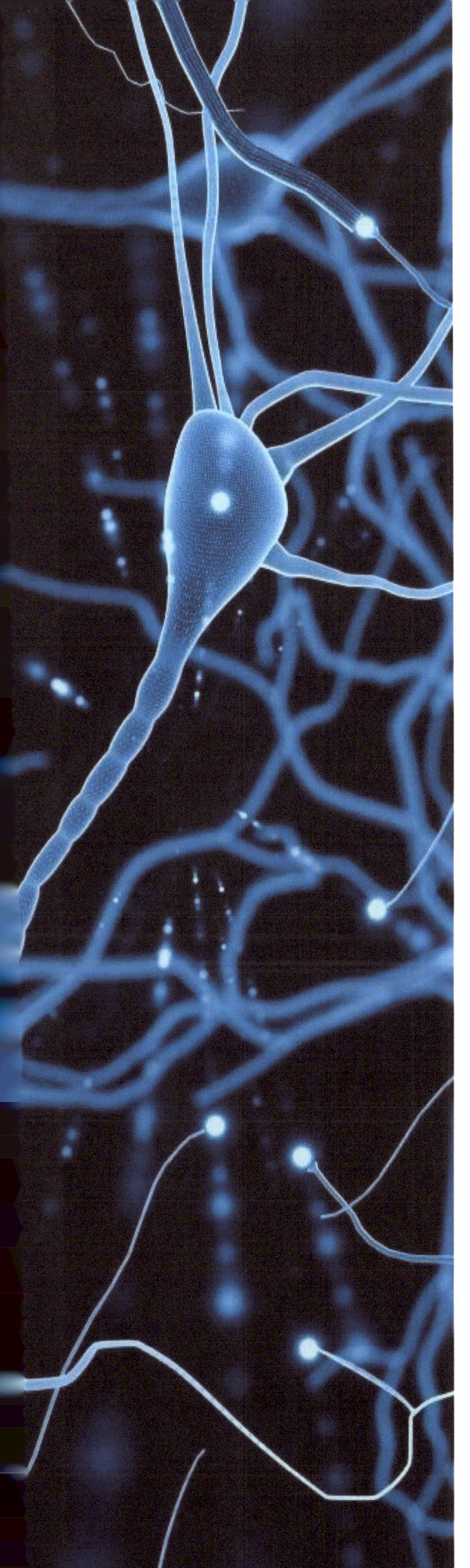

What Do You Remember?

By Cynthia Lim

Three months after my husband Perry's cardiac arrest and brain injury due to anoxia, I was still unsure of the extent of his brain damage and what remained of his former self. I knew he was never going to be able to resume his career as an attorney but I held out hope that his witty and loving self would return.

When he awoke from a two-week coma, he spent several months in acute-care hospitals in Los Angeles until he was transferred to a residential rehabilitation center in Pomona. There was no pattern to his behavior and no way of predicting what his state of mind would be when we visited. In his lucid moments, I saw glimpses of the former Perry, his sparkling eyes full of love, his Cheshire Cat smile with a sign of mischief, the arching of his brows and his deep, nasally voice. Whenever one of the attendants pointed to me and asked him, "Who's she?" he would always break into a smile and say the same thing: "My beautiful wife, Cynthia." But in his agitated moments, I didn't know who he was. There was a hardness in his eyes, a disconnection that made him appear as a stranger to me. He was lost in silence and unresponsive, frowning.

I hated the long drive to the rehabilitation center which often took more than an hour or sometimes up to ninety minutes during rush hour after work. During that long drive, I cried for my old life. I cried for my genial companion who was conversant, considerate, and made me laugh. I cried when I thought of our future, for the vacations still to be planned, for our dreams to grow old and retire together. I cried when he didn't recognize his favorite fly fishing reel.

Perry had loved fishing and had amassed a large collection of equipment. Before his expeditions, he would spend hours in the garage fussing with lines, rods and reels. He used to call me from work, excited about the latest purchase.

"Cyn, I just ordered this really nice Shimano fly fishing reel. I can use it for saltwater fly fishing. What do you think?"

"Sounds good to me," I said, not knowing the difference between a fly fishing reel for saltwater or freshwater, or why this one was so special.

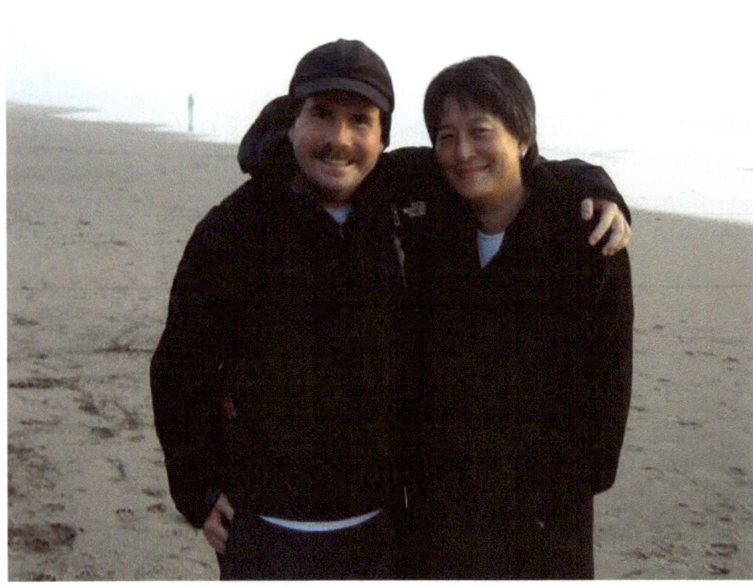
Cynthia and Perry Before His Injury

But after his brain injury, when I brought him that special reel at the rehabilitation center, he didn't recognize the purple felt bag. He took out the reel and ran his stubby fingers over the cut-out holes, then turned it over, his face puzzled.

"It's your special Shimano reel," I said. "Do you remember when you bought it and how excited you were?"

"No," he said, slowly turning it in his hands. With the weight he lost during his coma, the tops of his hands seemed more wrinkled and freckled. He put the Shimano reel on the desk.

"What about this one?" I asked, handing him another reel. He pulled the spool into place, then cranked it one turn.

"It's a spinning reel," he whispered, "for fishing with a lure or bait." He set it down on the desk, disinterested, then turned away. In that moment, it seemed that all hope was lost.

I felt like a widow but Perry wasn't dead. I was mourning the loss of someone who was still alive, albeit in a different form. And during those times, I longed for the comfort of religion. I thought of the healing prayer that Perry's cousins, both rabbi's, sang in Hebrew while he was in intensive care. I had squirmed when I heard the unfamiliar Hebrew words and didn't know if I should bow my head or look up. Perry was not observant as a Jew and my Chinese family never attended church. But the Hebrew phrases became comforting to me.

"Refaeinu Adonay V'Nerafeh, Hosheeinu v'nerasheinu kee Tehilateinu Atah, Heal us, oh God, and we shall be healed," I would sing to myself when I left the hospital in the evenings. Something about the cadence and melody resonated with me. I felt a sense of spirituality, a connection with an ancient tradition. And now, mourning for the old Perry and our old life, I longed for a formal ritual, a way to say goodbye to his former self. I wanted to sing a liturgy at a Catholic funeral mass, recite Kaddish in Hebrew, receive visitors while sitting Shiva or light incense and pray in his memory in a Buddhist temple.

I wondered if I could adapt to the new Perry and love him in the same way. I thought about what still remained to love and how bad it would have to get for me to stop loving him. What remained of a marriage if shared memories were lost? In most brain injury cases, short-term memory was the first to go, whereas long-term memory generally stayed intact. Memories that occurred right before the event were usually lost. I quizzed him on what he could remember.

"Do you remember our trip to Prague and Vienna?" I asked. We had gone there for spring break, three months before his heart attack.

"Not really," he said.

"How about your fishing trip to La Paz?" He had taken that trip a month before his heart attack with Paul, our younger son and our neighbor, Manny.

"Not really."

"What about Zack's graduation?" Our older son's high school graduation occurred the week before his heart attack.

He looked at me without a hint of recognition.

"What do you remember?" I asked.

"I remember going to law school and working really hard. I remember taking the bar exam and passing. I remember my law firm," he said, his voice fading to a whisper. "I remember how much I love you."

Meet Cynthia Lim

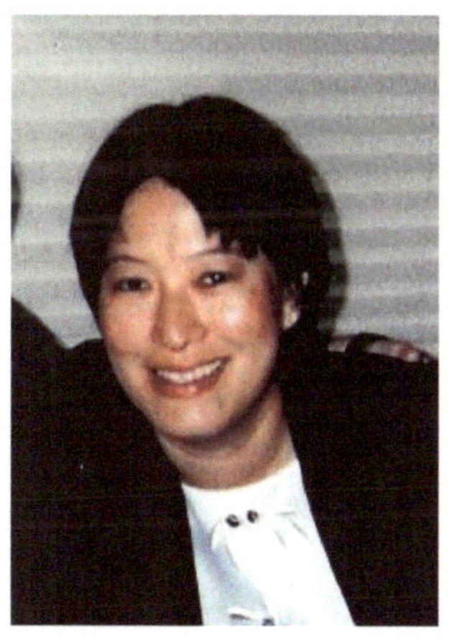

Cynthia Lim grew up in Salinas, California. She holds a BA in Experimental Psychology from UC Santa Barbara, a Masters in Social Work from UC Berkeley, and a doctorate in social welfare from UCLA, and had brief stints as a VISTA volunteer in Indianapolis, Indiana, and Boise, Idaho. She recently retired as the Executive Director for Data and Accountability for the Los Angeles Unified School District. She has lived in Los Angeles with her family for the past 30 years. For more info, visit cynthialimwriting.com.

> **"To be brave is to love someone unconditionally, without expecting anything in return."** *-Madonna*

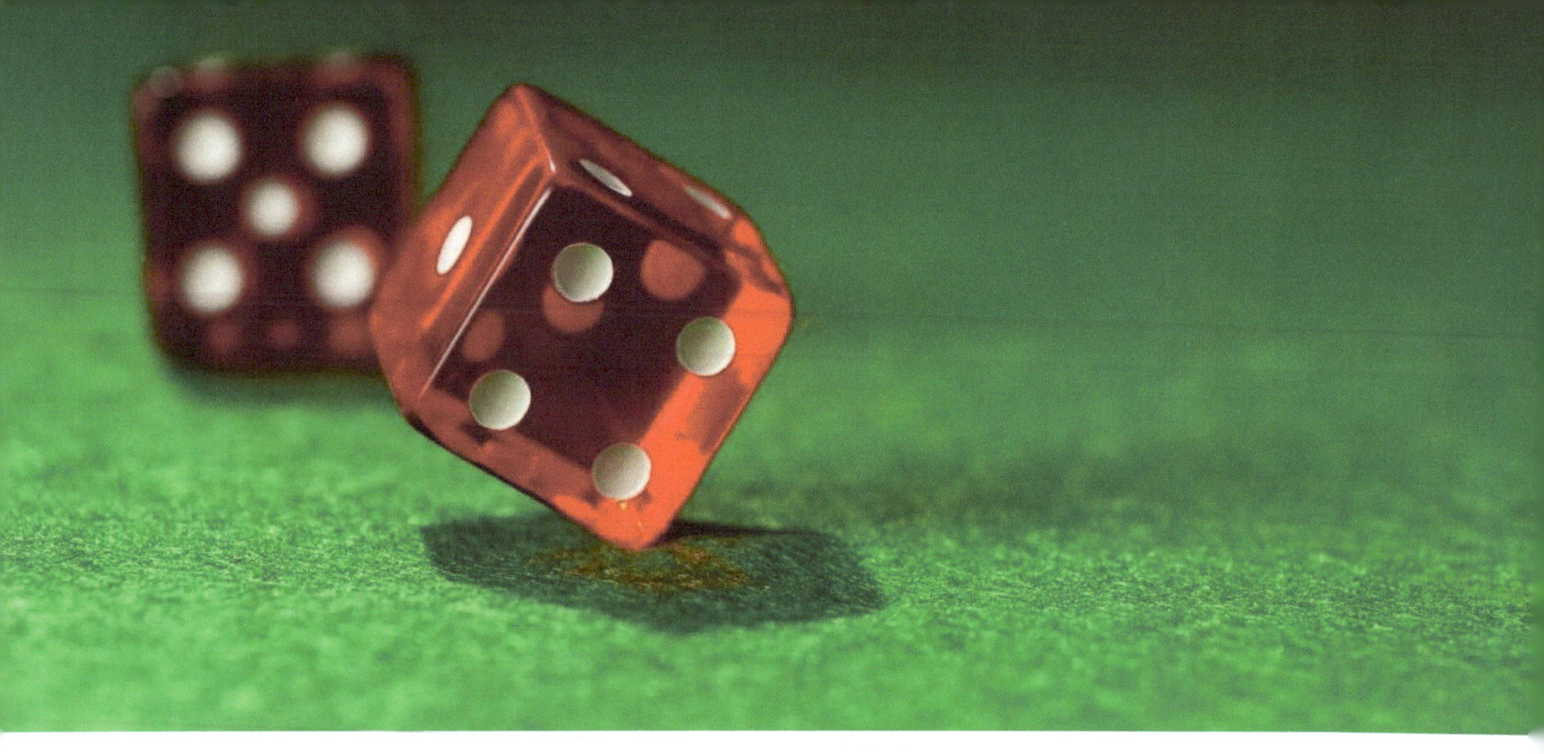

Beating the Odds

By Coral-Lynn Rubino

My TBI story begins back on May 22nd, 1999. At the time, I was just two-and-a-half year's old playing with my toys before I went to bed for the night. My younger brother, who was sixteen-months-old, was already in bed. My father went into the kitchen to grab a snack and I climbed up on the window sill of our second-story apartment and opened the window.

My father came back into the room, took me off of the window sill and closed the window before going back into the kitchen to finish what he was doing. When he went back into the kitchen, I returned to the window and opened it again. This time, I got startled and fell from that window, along with the screen, and landed on the pavement driveway below.

My mom wasn't home at the time of the accident, but when she saw the ambulance headed to the hospital, she knew something had happened.

My father screamed, which woke up my brother, and he ran down the stairs and outside where I laid motionless and lifeless. My father thought I was dead. The ambulance came and my father went to the hospital with me, while our neighbors watched my brother. My mom wasn't home at the time of the accident, but when she saw the ambulance headed to the hospital, she knew something had happened.

I was rushed to our local hospital and then transported to CHEO, which is the Children's Hospital of Eastern Ontario in Ottawa, Ontario. This is where I spent the next two months of my life, where my parents and family had no idea if I was going to survive and if I did what the outcome would be for my future. The left side of my brain was damaged, and over time the back of my left side brain died and diminished.

I was in a medically-induced coma for ten days and doctors told my parents that I probably wouldn't be able to walk by my third birthday. On Father's Day, I was able to come home from the hospital for the day and my grandparents and parents were crying with joy because they did not think I would ever come home.

When my third birthday came around I was walking by holding onto couches and tables for support, but I was walking. I started school two years after my accident occurred and had the supports I needed to be able to succeed in school.

When I was eight years old, I slipped and fell at a wave pool and received a concussion on the right side of my brain. After this, I was taken to the children's hospital for a week to recover.

Years after both accidents, I graduated from high school in 2014 at the age of seventeen. My schooling continued and I graduated from college and am currently working toward my degree from the University of Victoria.

Though I only have three-quarters of my brain alive, I've beaten all the odds that the doctors have given me. My only long-term deficits are having no use of my right hand and limited use of my right leg. My brain injury has not affected my intelligence at all.

Though I only have three-quarters of my brain alive, I've beaten all the odds that the doctors have given me.

Today, at 21 years old, I'm going into my fourth year of University and have so much to offer. I'm studying to become a Child and Youth Care Practitioner where I can provide support to children and youth who are struggling. My dream job is counseling in the mental health sector and nothing holds me back to follow this dream, or any dream.

My story is one of the successful ones because who knows, the outcome could have been a whole lot different.

Meet Coral-Lynn Rubino

Coral-Lynn Writes…

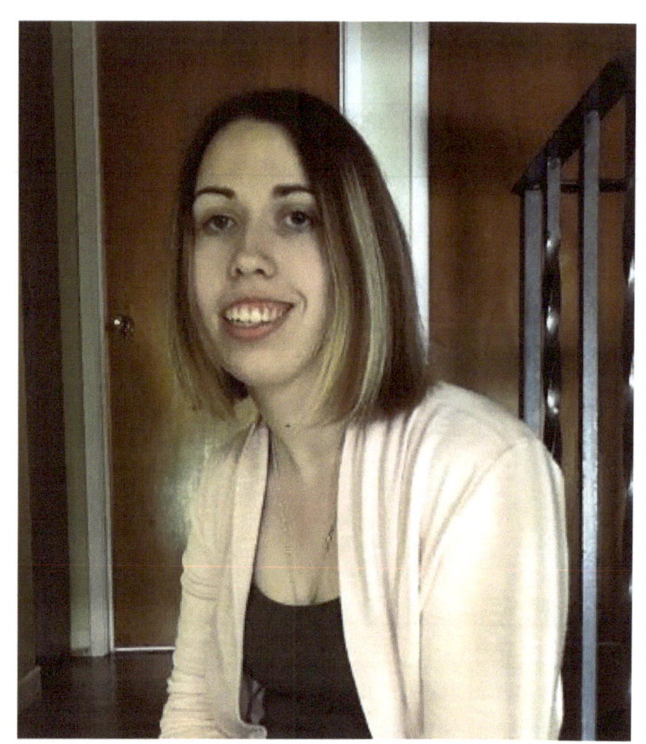

"I currently reside in Brockville Ontario, Canada which is on the St. Lawrence River and the border of the United States. I believe having grown up with my TBI has helped me reach my full potential because I do not have any memories before my accident. My grandparents said that before the accident I didn't tell them which hand I would be, but after my accident I was automatically left-handed due to the mobility in my right hand had gone.

Today at nineteen years post injury, I enjoy reading and writing in my spare time, but most importantly I focus on my studies as it takes me a little longer to complete, but I am able to succeed and get high marks. With having struggled with depression and anxiety I hope to one day publish something I wrote and to counsel children and youth."

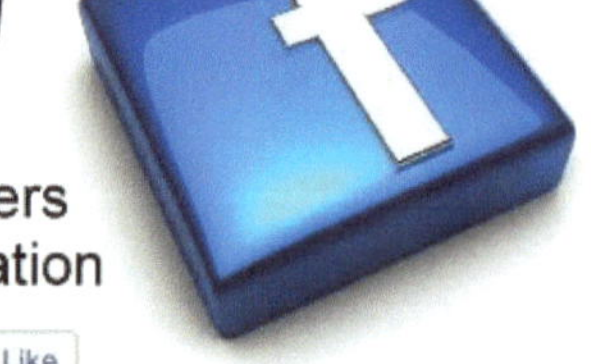

INTRODUCING THE NEW
dish FLEX PACK
Create Your Own TV Package

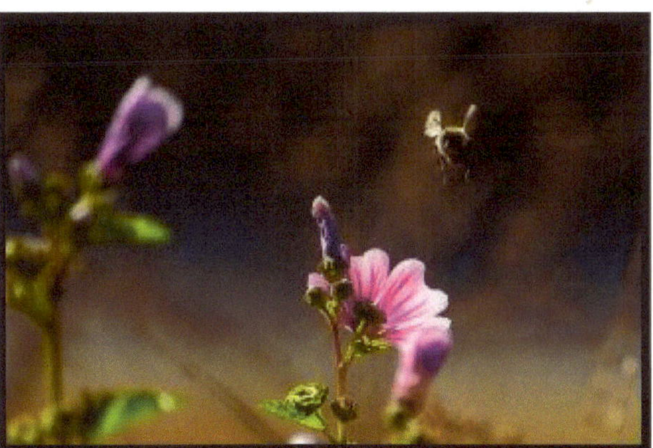

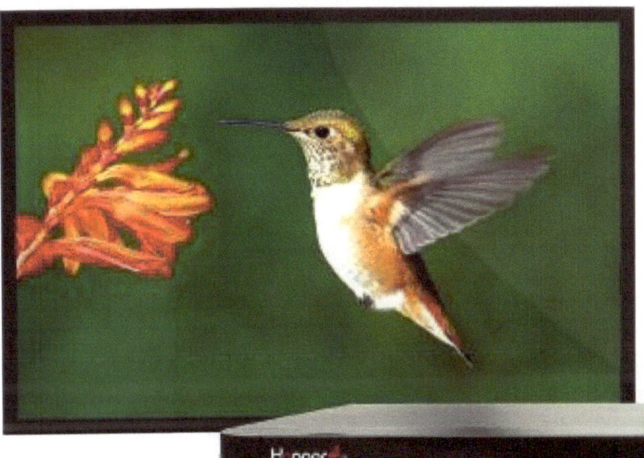

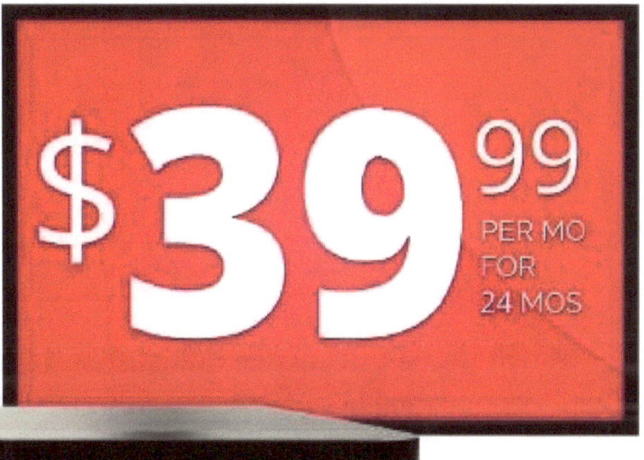

Free Streaming

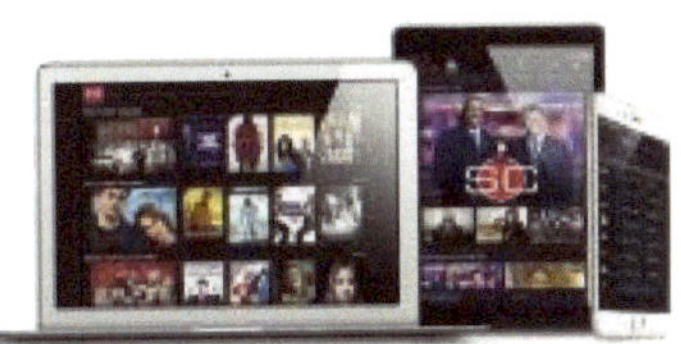

+

Free Installation

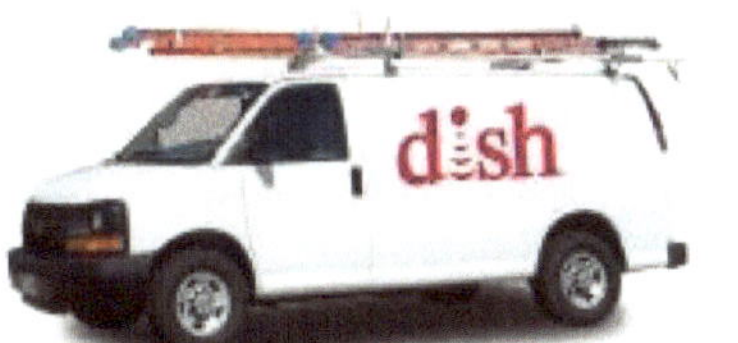

+

Add Internet

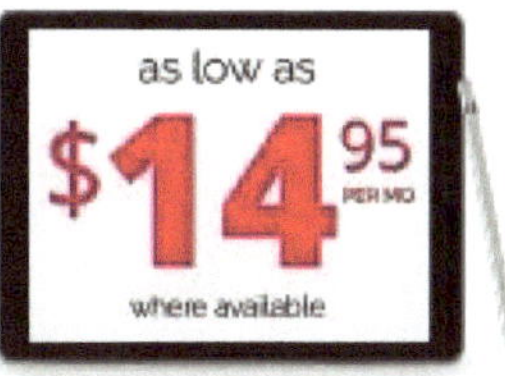

Call 1-800-391-1328

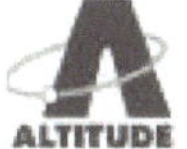

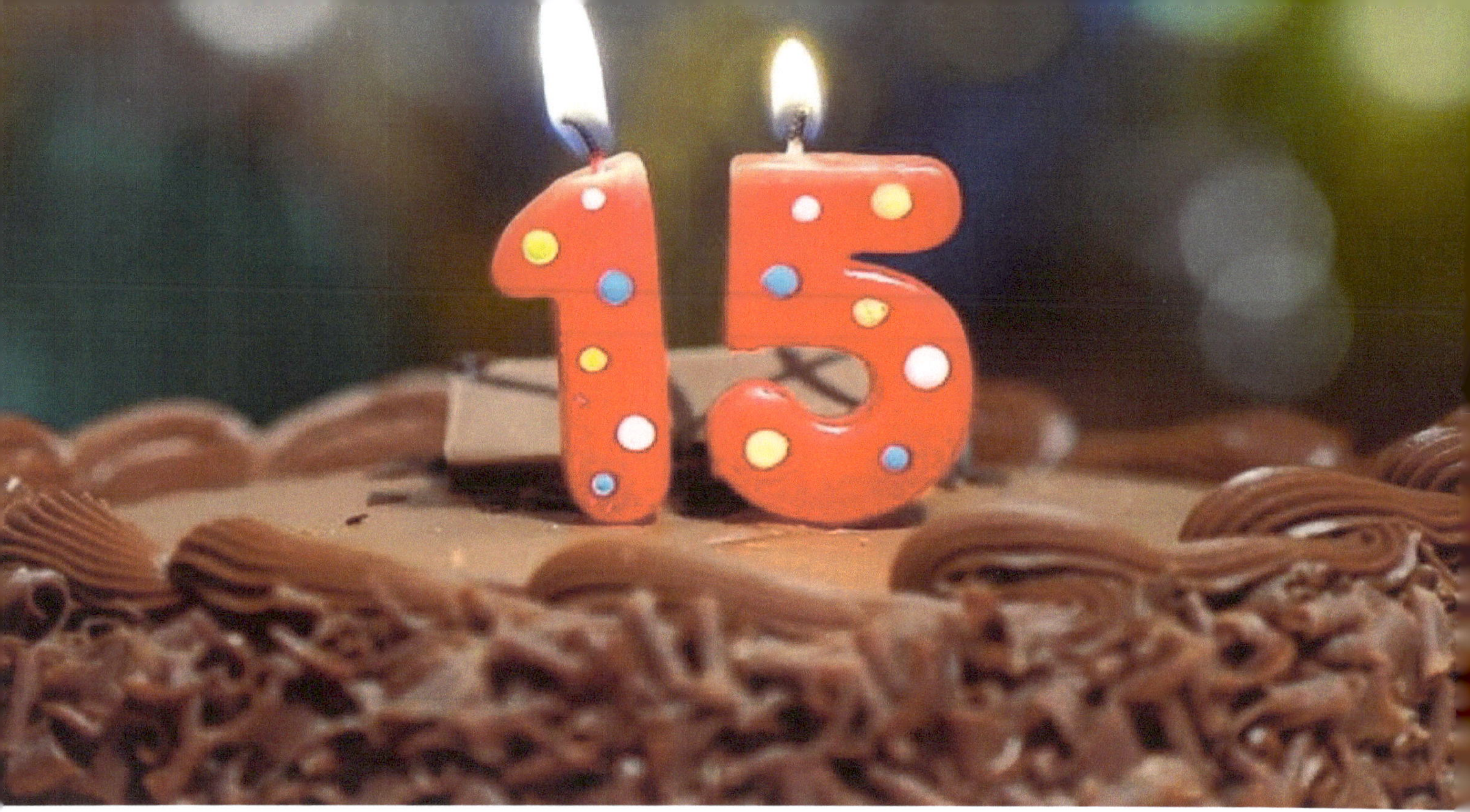

Fifteen Years Out

By Ric Johnson

October 18th will be the fifteen-year anniversary of my brainday. I refuse to call it a birthday. Sometimes, I think there is nothing about recovering from a traumatic brain injury that I have not seen or felt before. However, any day, any event can tell me I have not seen everything. When talking about recovering from a traumatic brain injury I am, of course, only talking about my recovery. What other survivors are going through may be very close to my experiences, but my difficulties are differently mine.

I am fortunate as I do not have any "major" medical issues, so my real difficulties are fatigue, speech, and balance. Fatigue seems to be the kicker. Regardless of what I am doing, after 45-60 minutes, I need a break. Without taking a break, anything can go south.

What about general day-to-day tasks like the grocery store? Before I leave home, I write a list of items to buy, ordered by aisle. So here I am at the grocery store. On the first aisle are the fruit and blueberries that are on my list. I cannot just grab any container, I have to look at them carefully.

Amount, check. Color, check. Expiration date, check. Into my grocery cart they go.

Next item, bananas… and on and on with the fresh fruit list I go.
Next aisle? Produce. First is sweet potatoes - Color, check. Size, check. Amount, check.

I'll stop reading my full grocery list, because I'm sure you get the picture. That is how trips to the grocery store go for me most of the time. What could happen that would change my regular grocery experience? The store reorganized their aisles but didn't change the signs hanging above the aisles. After many attempts trying to find napkins, I needed to ask a clerk.

> With aphasia, everything can go wrong. If you say nachos instead of napkins, they send you to the wrong aisle.

What could go wrong?

With aphasia, everything can go wrong. If you say nachos instead of napkins, they send you to the wrong aisle. After looking at everything in the snacks aisle, I cursed aphasia because it knew that napkins and nachos both start with the letter N. This fooled my brain into thinking I was saying napkins, even though it had me say nachos. I needed to say napkins multiple times under my breath before I asked another clerk.

A few weeks ago, I had planned on taking a vacation. Before getting out-of-town, I made my to-do list of items needing my attention. The first item was to read my to-do-list.

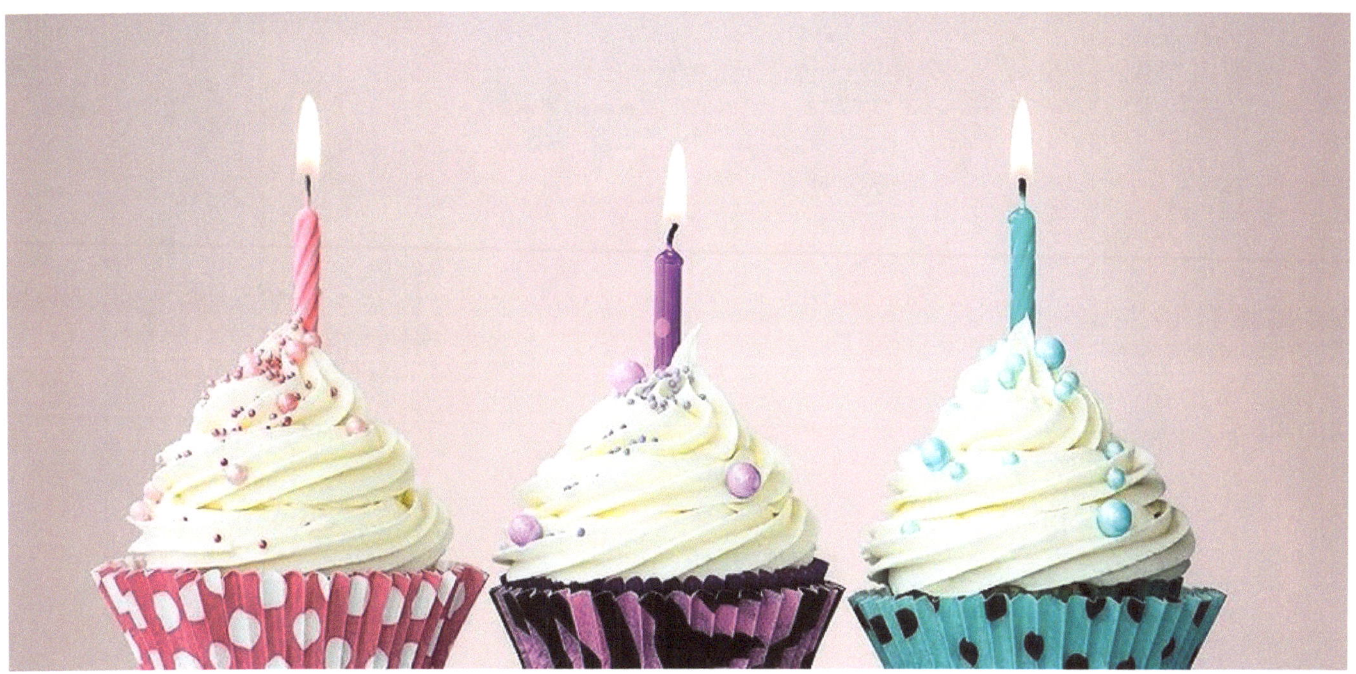

Task 1: change the cat litter boxes. Don't have "new" cat litter at home so will need to go to a store to buy.

What's task 2? Vacuum the house. Not a problem, so I'll do that first, then change the litter boxes.

Task 3? Check and maybe clean out the traps for the kitchen sink. OK, let's re-number that list. kitchen sink first, then vacuum, then litter boxes.

I didn't mention that balance needs to be addressed as well. Falling and hitting my head again triggers my PTSD, so when walking up and down stairs to finish task 1 and 2 above, my eyes are glued to my feet. Actually, when walking anywhere anytime, looking at the floor, sidewalk, yard and my feet, grounds me.

Fatigue is the main key of my daily existence. Total time for tasks above was about four hours. Regardless of the time spent and work done, my brain worked harder than any other part of my body. My brain needs quiet time to refocus and recharge.

Another part of working and finishing those tasks is staying focused. It is so easy to get distracted; I know that I cannot start thinking about anything else. Easier said than done, but when I stay focused on the task, everything seems to fit in place.

After fifteen years of practice, practice, practice I still need to tell myself the best is yet to come.

This article has taken me over five hours to write, and it's time to submit. As soon as I click the "send" button, I'll find my favorite comfy chair and take a nap.

Meet Ric Johnson

Ric Johnson is a husband, father, grandfather and a traumatic brain injury survivor of fifteen years. Ric is also a member of the Speaker Bureau for the Minnesota Brain Injury Alliance, and facilitator for The Courage Kenny Brain Injury Support Group.

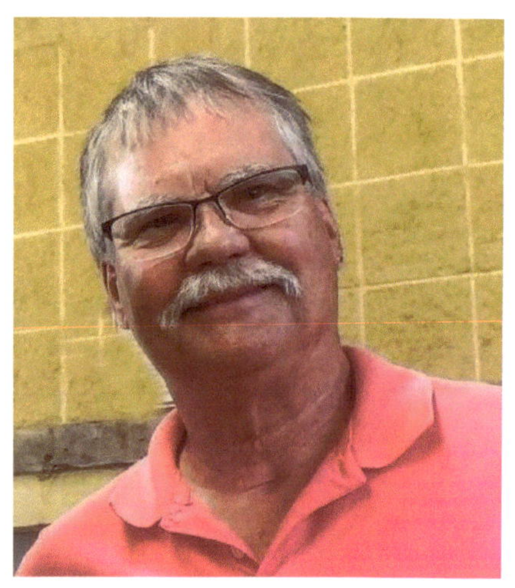

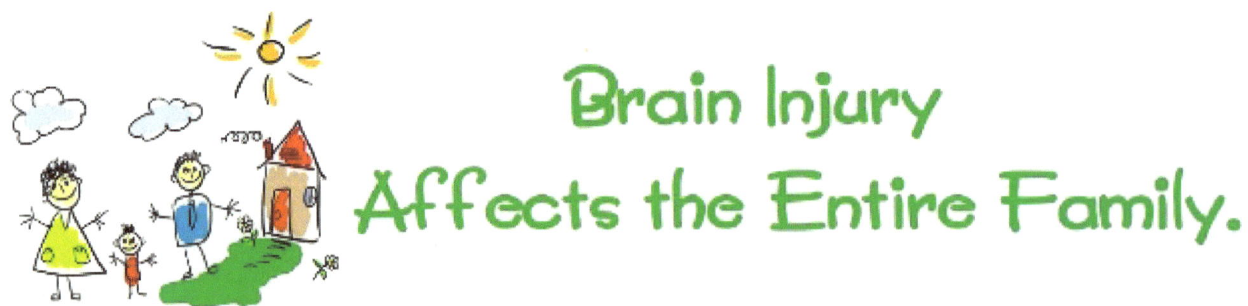

A Help Button Should Go Where You Go!

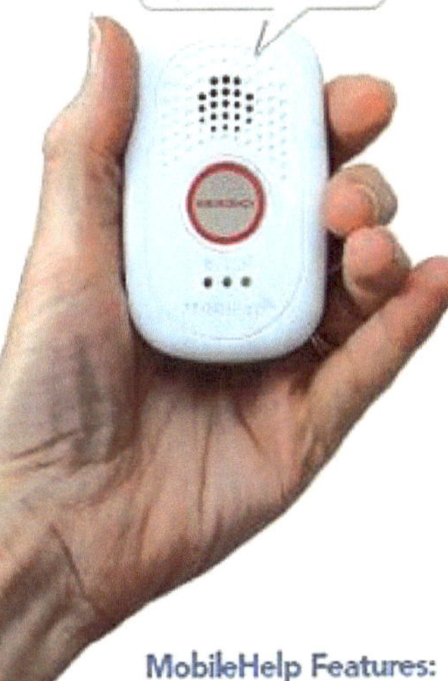

To be truly independent your personal emergency device needs to work on the go.

MobileHelp® allows you to summon emergency help 24 hours a day, 365 days a year by simply pressing your personal help button. Unlike traditional systems that only work inside your home, MobileHelp's medical alert system extends help beyond the home. Now you can participate in all your favorite activities such as gardening, taking walks, shopping and traveling all with the peace of mind of having a personal medical alert system with you. MobileHelp, the "on-the-go" help button, is powered by one of the nation's largest cellular networks, so there's virtually no limit to your help button's range.* With our GPS feature activated, we can send help to you, even when you can't talk or tell us where you are.

No landline? No Problem! While traditional medical alert systems require a landline, with MobileHelp's system, a landline is not necessary. Whether you are home or away from home, a simple press of your help button activates your system, providing the central station with your information and location. Our trained emergency operators will know who you are and where you are located.

If you're one of the millions of people that have waited for a medical alert service because it didn't fit your lifestyle, or settled for a traditional system even though it only worked in the home, then we welcome you to try MobileHelp. Experience peace of mind in the home or on the go.

MobileHelp Features:

- Simple one-button operation
- Affordable service
- Amplified 2-way voice communication
- 24/7/365 access to U.S. based operators
- GPS location detection
- Available Nationwide

As seen on:

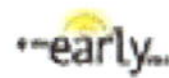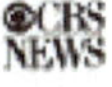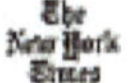

Optional Fall Button™

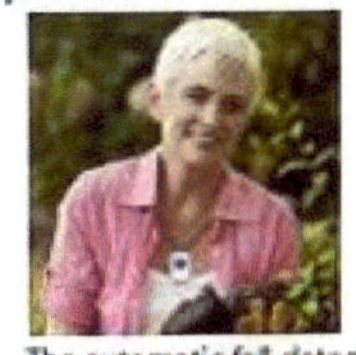

The automatic fall detect pendant that works **WHERE YOU GO!**

Unlike 'stay-at-home' emergency systems MobileHelp protects you:		
Places where your Help Button will work	MobileHelp	Traditional Help Buttons
Home	✓	✓
On a Walk	✓	✗
On Vacation	✓	✗
At the Park	✓	✗
Shopping	✓	✗

Order Now & Receive a FREE Lockbox!

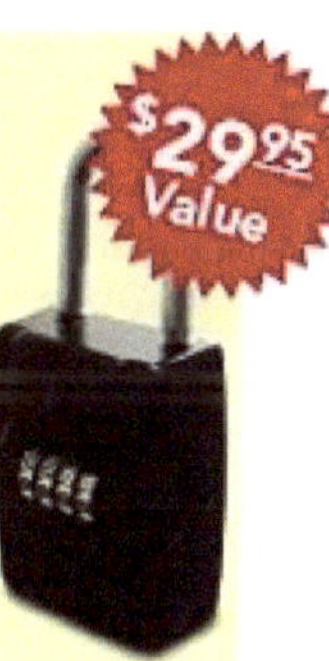

Place your door key in this box so that emergency personnel can get help to you even faster.

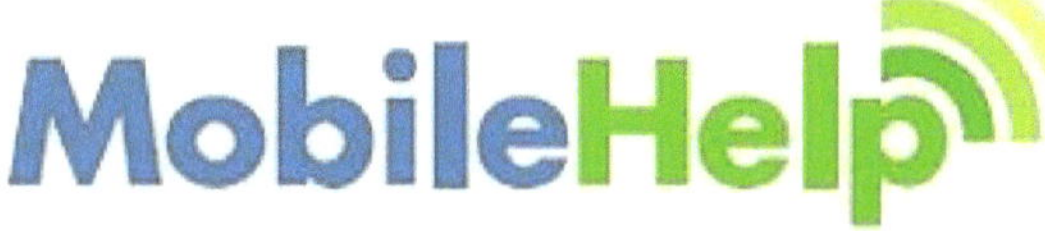

1-800-371-2132

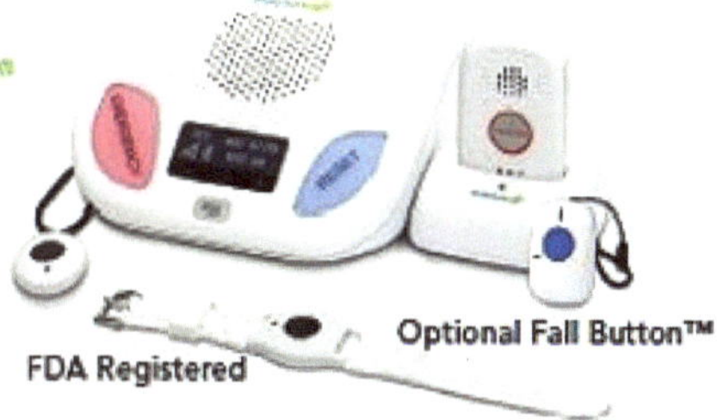

FDA Registered

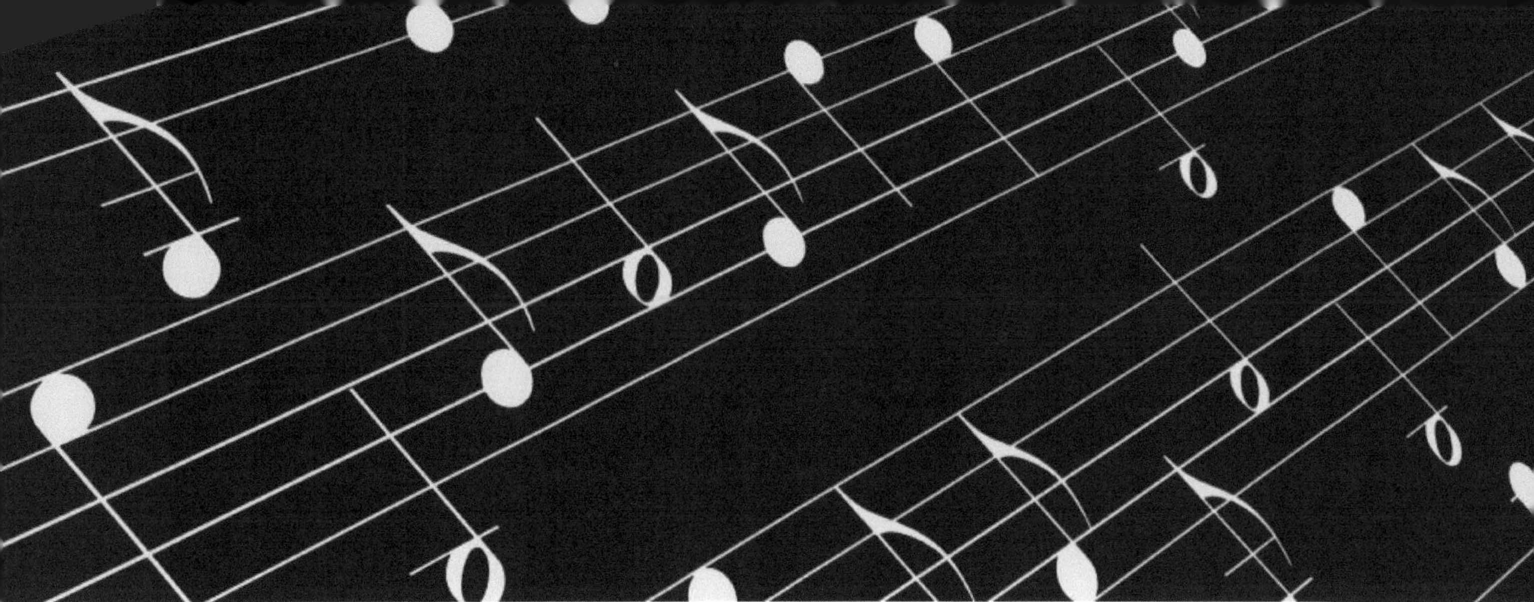

Back to Where I Once Belonged

By Lisa Yee

Music was a big part of my life growing up—piano lessons, church choir, school band, theater—not to mention the songs playing nonstop in my head. That internal soundtrack is still going, but now I also have the fun lack of decorum that comes with traumatic brain injury, so I hum or sing along to my heart's content, where appropriate … usually.

By far my favorite is Beatles music. I'd gotten way, way into the group when I was in eighth grade, and I'm only 51. It shames me to say that it was John Lennon's murder on Dec. 8, 1980, that sparked my interest in the Fab Four, but I was a little young to be a first-generation fan.

In college, this guy Ted, who would go on to become my husband, learned I had an encyclopedic knowledge of All Things Beatles. Even with other music, he noticed my lyrical memory was weirdly spot-on, even for songs I'd only heard coming from my siblings' stereos or seen in songbooks. After 1993, when our daughter was born, I learned lots of "Barney & Friends" songs, sang her lullabies and helped her master the state capitals by singing them.

> I emerged from a coma with moderate TBI and multiple broken bones and internal injuries, lucky to be alive.

The Accident came years later, in September 2008. I emerged from a coma with moderate TBI and multiple broken bones and internal injuries, lucky to be alive. As cool as it would have been, though, I didn't "wake up to the sound of music," as in "Let It Be," Paul McCartney's ode to his mother. According to Ted, I once awoke in the hospital saying, in a robotic voice, "ERR-or. ERR-or," and

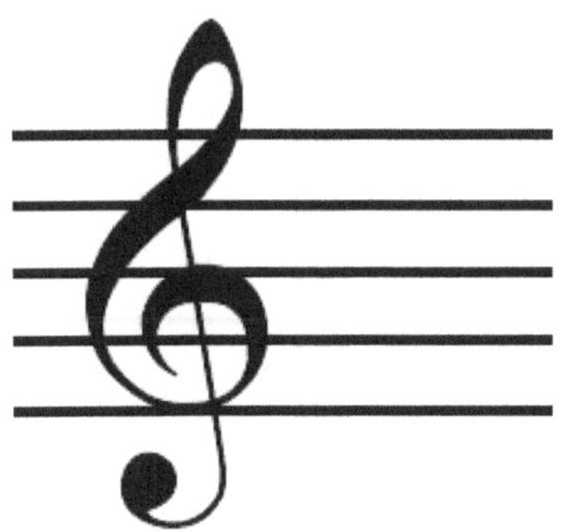

It was as if my brain needed a nudge and then muscle memory took over.

something like "01010101010." I guess my brain was a computer, resetting itself. Or maybe that came from a repressed edition of "Lost in Space."

But my soundtrack wouldn't be silenced. I must have gotten pretty enthusiastic singing around the house and in public. One Christmas, Ted gave me an electronic keyboard, pointing out that its settings included Grand Piano. I'll assume this gift was intended to bring me joy and enhance my brain's recovery, not to confine my musical stylings to the home. I didn't use the keyboard much for a long time. The truth is, it came with a bunch of instructions and music lessons, and I got frustrated easily. Also, I never was good at sight-reading, and the brain injury had messed with my vision. So the keyboard sat dormant for a while.

Then, on a visit back home, I was at the upright piano complaining that I couldn't remember how to play Lennon's "Imagine." My brother, the only one of us with any real piano-playing chops, showed me a bit of the right-hand part of the introduction, and something in my head went "Boom!" Days later, I started messing with that snippet of the intro on my own keyboard. Suddenly, I remembered the verses, the bridge, and the chorus!

There have been a bunch of musical revelations since then, including total recall of "Let It Be" and "Hey Jude." It was as if my brain needed a nudge and then muscle memory took over. This sort of thing happened again when a friend and former colleague, who posts a musical-clip-of-the-day on Facebook, shared a Scott Joplin rag that stopped me in my tracks. I sat down at the keyboard and, little by little, played "The Entertainer." When I joyfully thanked him for the mental boost, he said it had been a different Joplin number!

I've been reading "Musicophilia: Tales of Music and the Brain" by the late Dr. Oliver Sacks. You may recall Sacks as the author of "Awakenings," later a movie starring Robin Williams, about patients brought out of catatonic states with an experimental drug. In "Musicophilia," Sacks writes of "procedural memories" or "fixed action patterns" (muscle memory?) in the making of music. He says such patterns—as opposed to "episodic memory," or the recall of events—can sometimes be unaffected by amnesia.

Another brain-music connection I wanted to explore was how it could be that, post-TBI, I seem to have gained an understanding of harmony. I've always had a hard time sight-reading, unless I'm playing only the right-hand, or treble clef, part—the melody, in other words. But for me, reading the treble and bass (harmony) notes at same time, all while making sure my fingers are on the right keys, is too much multitasking. To cope, I usually end up memorizing the left-hand part, and memorization isn't so easy these days.

Fortunately, I've always been able to tap out melodies by ear. In the past couple of years, I've found I can incorporate my own harmony just by adding notes that sound right; I can sense what works and what doesn't. When I've figured out a few bars, I scribble down the notes—F, G and so on—even though I don't have the patience to put them all in note form on musical staff paper.

"Musicophilia" doesn't address my question about harmony, but Sacks does say that with temporal lobe seizures (the type to which I have been prone), medical literature lists "many accounts of the onset of musical or artistic inclinations." He describes a man whose heart stopped briefly in 1994 when he was struck by lightning. After a few weeks of memory problems and a neurological check, he felt well enough to return to work. Soon he was overcome by a desire for piano music—first to listen, then to play and then to compose. Mind you, this patient had no musical talent before.

I'll have to throw in some other brain research here to explain a more recent musical experience. After taking a tumble down the basement stairs earlier this year—a laundry/stupidity-related accident, not a seizure—I was mostly confined to the couch for two months. I was bored. I was angry. I read more news and social media than usual, which did not help. Eventually, deprived of my usual obsessive amount of physical activity, I decided to make my brain useful and focus on my keyboard.

I was practicing some song or another when a waltz I used to play as a kid magically filled my head. After several false starts, I remembered. By the time I was finished, I knew what this song was but not the title.

Now, buckle up, folks, because this is about to get weird: I closed my eyes and mentally "went" to Mom and Dad's piano bench, opened it and took out the red songbook that I suddenly remembered. I looked up the title. Ladies and gentlemen, I tell you, that's how I remembered "The Irene Waltz."

Seatbelts still fastened? There's more. Mom died in 2007, less than a year before The Accident. I still don't remember the funeral, but I must have known she was gone, because I asked about her from my hospital bed. Though my memory has improved in the past few years—thanks to better neurological care—years of gaps remain. After thinking, writing and thinking some more about the "Irene Waltz" experience, I've come to feel in my heart that Mom was somehow giving me a gift.

Studies have shown that music from specific time periods can bring back vivid memories. You can see this for yourself in the 2014 documentary "Alive Inside: A Story of Music and Memory," a clip of which had already gone viral in 2012. In it, Henry, a dementia patient and 10-year nursing home resident, is described as "unresponsive and almost unalive" until he is given an iPod with headphones that let him hear music from his youth. When a Cab Calloway song begins, he visibly "comes alive," singing along, talking, and keeping the beat.

I'd stumbled upon the film clip on the Internet and was trying to identify the doctor being interviewed. Just as I was about to give up on quoting him, I looked down at the author photo on the cover of "Musicophilia," the book that my own neurologist—Dr. Elizabeth Gerard of Chicago—had recommended when I told her I was writing this. The man in the movie clip and on the book cover were one and the same: Oliver Sacks!

"Music," he says in the book, "can animate, organize and bring a sense of identity back to people who are 'out of it.' Music will bring them back 'into it,' back into their own personhood, their own memories and their own autobiographies."

Or as in my case, back to where they once belonged.

Meet Lisa Yee

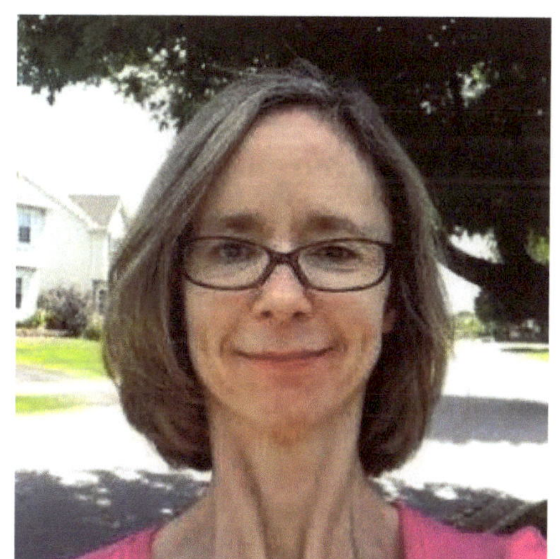

Lisa Yee of suburban Chicago suffered a traumatic brain injury/epilepsy in a 2008 car accident. Before her injury, she had been a newspaper editor for two decades after graduating from the Indiana University School of Journalism. It was there she met her husband, Ted. They have a daughter, Megan, of Chicago.

Post TBI, Lisa became certified as a yoga instructor and now volunteers teaching yoga at a women's shelter and a veteran's center.

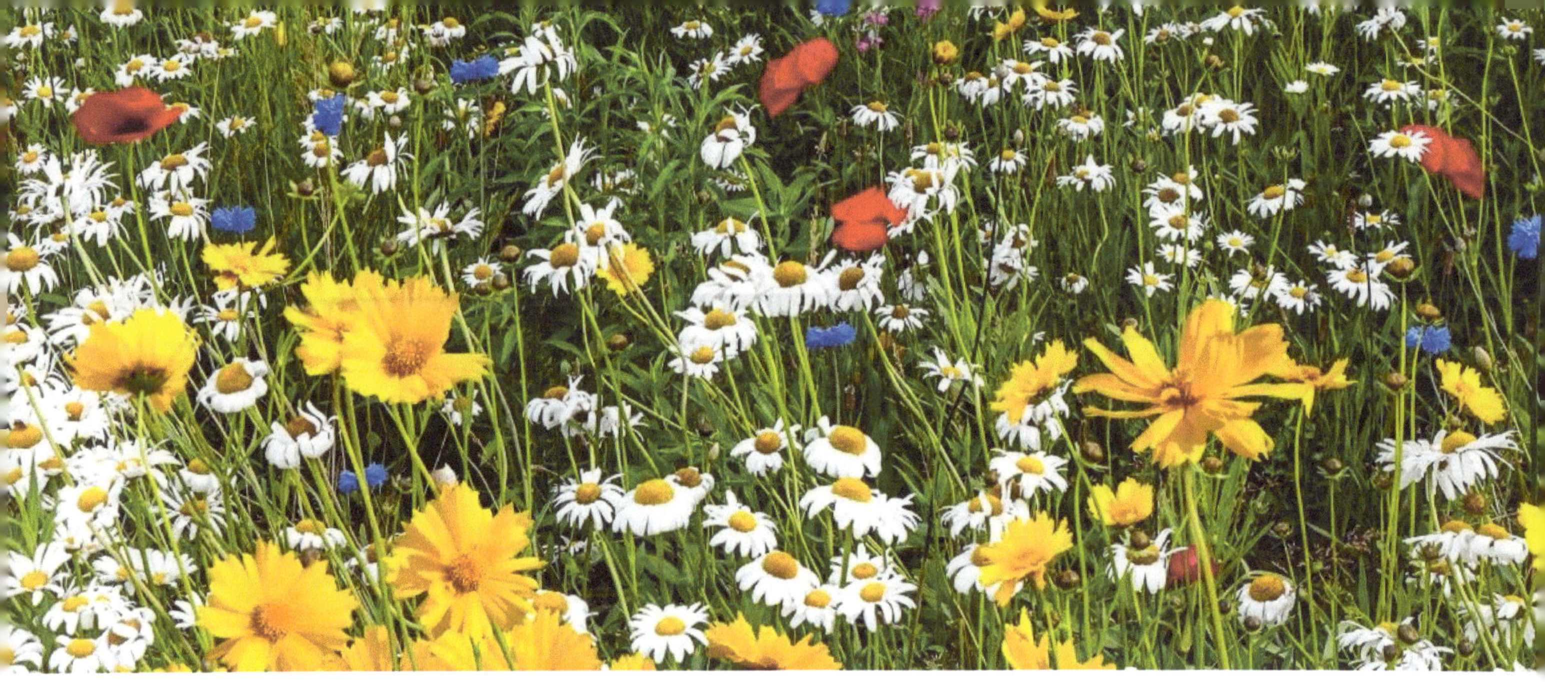

For the Love of a Dog

By Michelle Bartlett

It has been a year since I lost my beloved cocker spaniel Molly. Molly was twelve-years-old when I lost her from heart disease.

The first time I saw Molly, she was two-weeks-old and hadn't even opened her eyes yet. It had only been a little over a year since my brain injury. She immediately cuddled close to my heart and fell fast asleep. I knew I had found my heart dog.

Molly remained with her mother until she was properly weaned and allowed to leave. I visited her and her sisters on a regular basis, and it was always a joy to see how she was thriving and growing into a beautiful baby.

Everyone who met Molly immediately fell in love with her.

When Molly was a puppy she was mischievous, curious, and adventurous. I could return from a doctor's appointment to find that she had taken a $100.00 bill from my mom's purse and proceeded to eat most

> The first time I saw Molly, she was two-weeks-old and hadn't even opened her eyes yet. It had only been a little over a year since my brain injury.

of it, or she would chase a few birds or a squirrel that happened to get a little too close to her. Playing in the snow was something she enjoyed until the last few years of her life.

Molly was my unofficial emotional support dog.

We travelled across Canada and back together. She even went to a Bon Jovi concert with me. We dipped our toes in the cold glacier water of the Rocky Mountains on the west coast and the warm Atlantic Ocean on the east coast.

We needed each other. We loved each other unconditionally.

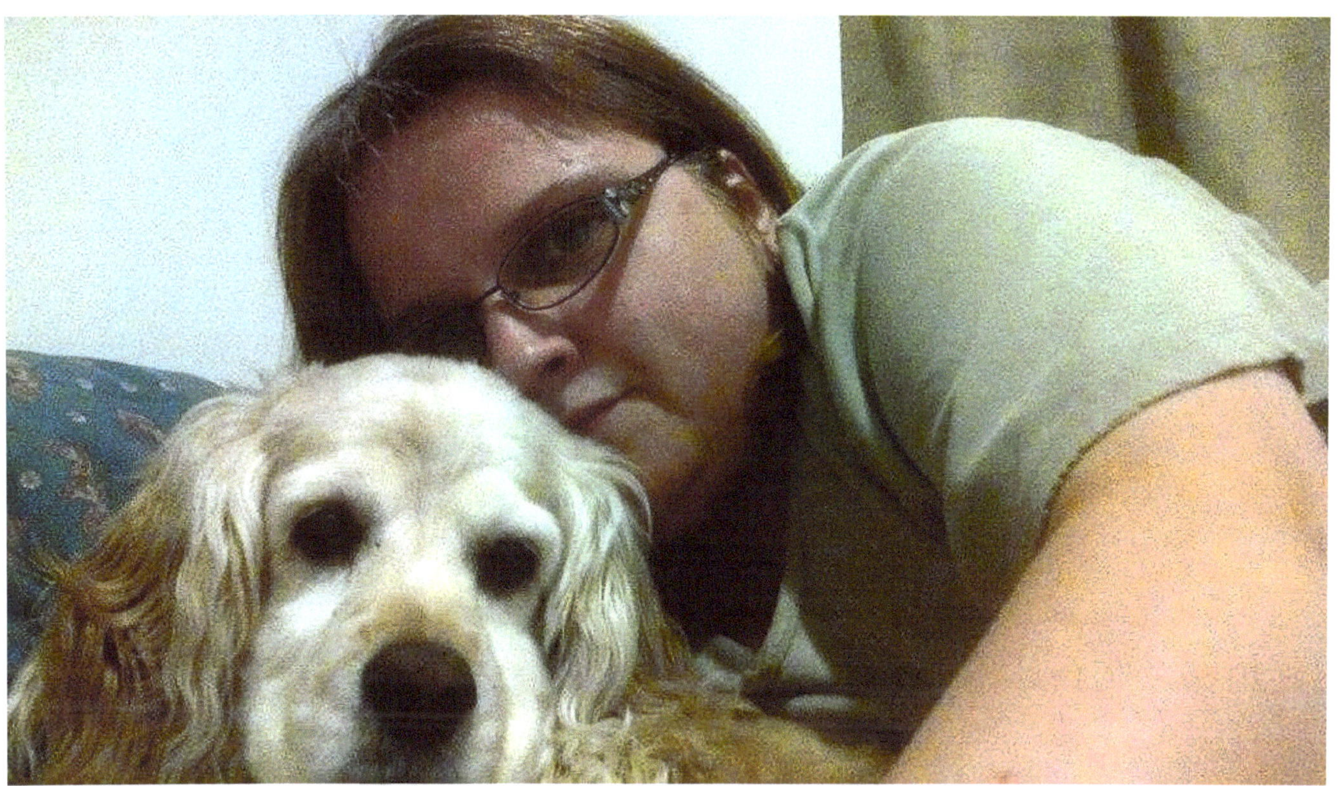

Michelle and Her Beloved Dog Molly

The love of a dog, or any animal, after a brain injury is hard to explain. I had dogs throughout most of my life but the connection I had with Molly was much different than any of my other dogs.

I was more emotional after my brain injury and Molly calmed me. Stress from very minor daily activities followed me day to day. I needed routines. Molly needed routines. We had a win-win situation.

Molly was literally a life-saver in more ways than one. She wasn't quite a year old and our house caught fire in the middle of the night. Molly woke up my ex-husband and I before the smoke alarms went off and we were able to escape safely. Unfortunately, there had been too much damage done to save the house.

Shortly after the house fire, we moved to the west coast of Canada to re-start our lives. My ex-husband was a truck driver and was away from home most of the time.

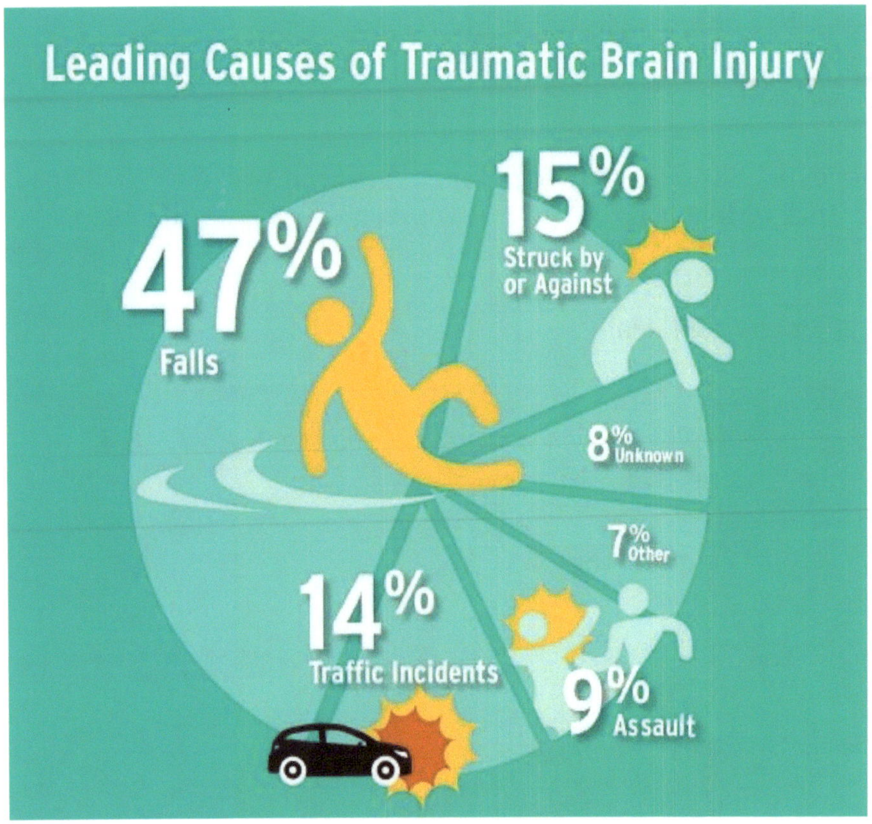

After my brain injury, my eyesight was affected, and my vision was comprised. I became scared of driving or trying anything new that involved focusing. Eye fatigue was real and the headaches followed if I pushed too hard.

Quickly, I realized that Molly and I needed a social life. So, I began exploring the town we lived in. It was slow in the beginning. We did meet people: other brain injury survivors, other dog lovers, spouses of truck drivers. It wasn't easy, but I saw the joy and improvement in the quality of both of our lives, so I kept going and improving.

My mom was in the twilight years of her life. She moved from the east coast to the west coast and lived with us the last few years of her life. Mom, Molly and I were so close and so much alike in personalities.

The year after Mom passed away, my husband and I decided to separate and Molly and I had our own little apartment on the west coast. It was the first time I had lived on my own since my brain injury. I wasn't sure if I had the skills I needed. I did.

The rest of my family wanted Molly and I to return to the east coast a few years later. I worried about the impact it would have on Molly. She spent the majority of her life on the west coast. The cold arctic air in the winter didn't bother her. She actually loved it. In the summer she would sit on the deck for hours watching for wildlife, or her friends. She loved life. It was infectious.

Molly and I moved back east and got an apartment and a car. After the initial transitional phase, we were settling in and rebuilding our lives. Molly gained new friends. She saw places that she hadn't seen since she was a puppy.

On a yearly check up to the vet, I was told that Molly had a heart problem but it was nothing to be concerned about. She was healthy and active but it needed to be monitored. Honestly, I never even gave it a second thought. I had my heart dog, my emotional support. I blocked any negative thoughts or feelings.

Soon it became unavoidable that Molly did indeed have a serious heart problem. She declined rapidly.

The hardest thing I have done since my injury was to say "Good-Bye" to my heart dog. It was the right thing to do.

Molly still is with me. She is in my heart, my memories and her picture is in a locket around my neck.

It is amazing to think that my whole journey was all for the love of a dog.

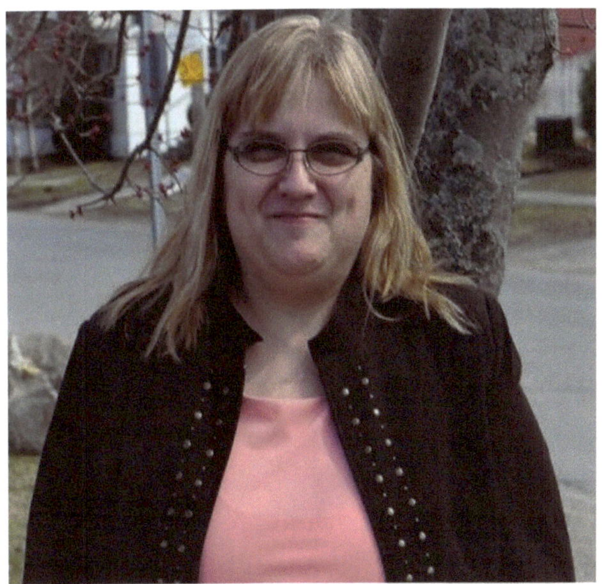

Meet Michelle Bartlett

Michelle had a severe anoxic brain injury in 2004, two days after open heart surgery in New Brunswick, Canada. The doctors pronounced her brain dead with no hope of survival, but after almost two weeks in a deep coma she started to regain consciousness. Michelle has spent the last fourteen years regaining ground. She received the Award of Merit from Brain Injury Canada in 2016 for her volunteer and advocacy work. Currently, Michelle resides in St. David Ridge New Brunswick. She plans to continue her advocacy and volunteer work.

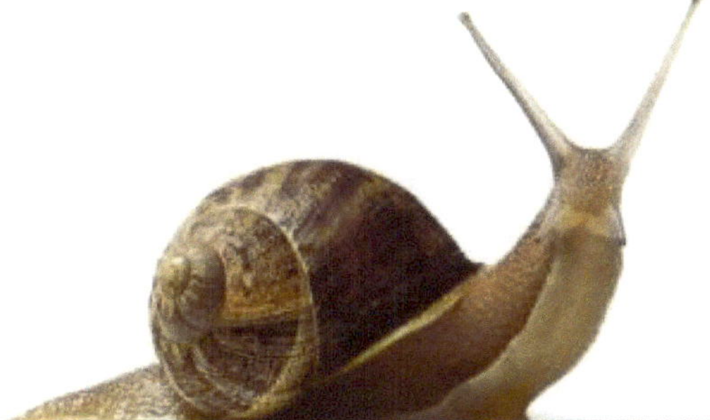

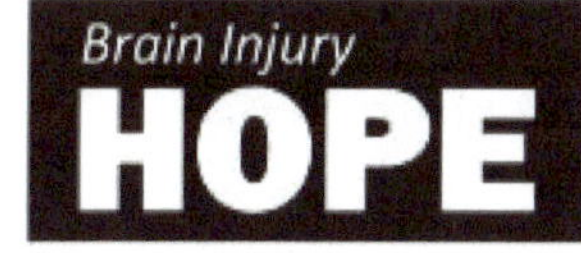

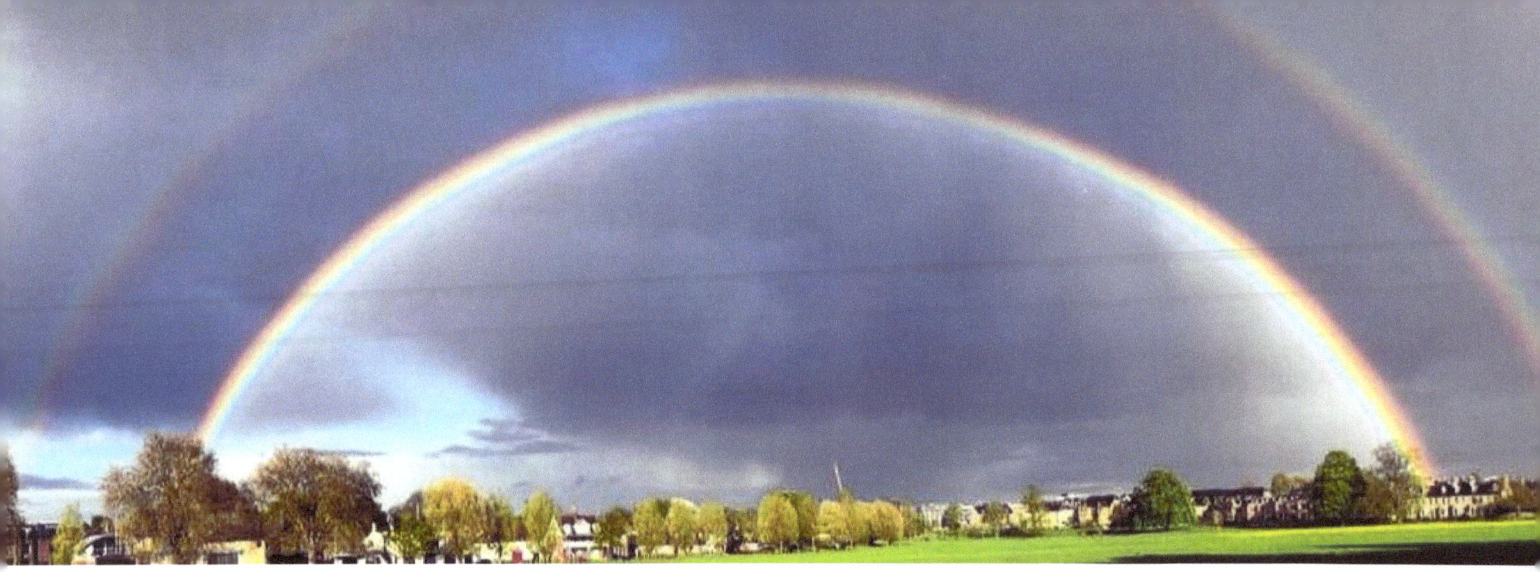

A Mother's Journey
By Norma Myers

Watching our children grow up with great anticipation of what's to come is a natural part of parenting. With pom-poms in hand, we celebrate every milestone. We experience butterflies when the big learner's permit day arrives. When we drop our baby off at college, we cry like babies ourselves! And low and behold the day arrives when we find ourselves attempting to embrace the long anticipated empty nest chapter. Dads tend to adjust more easily (*and eagerly*) to the empty nest chapter than Moms do. Go figure! All of these stages are normal for parents while learning to let go.

Three years ago, I found out what's not a normal stage of letting go. I was faced with prematurely saying goodbye to my first-born son at the fragile age of twenty-six while watching my other son fight for his life. Our sons Aaron and Steven were in a fatal car accident. Aaron didn't survive. Steven sustained a severe Traumatic Brain Injury (TBI) and was not expected to live.

Bending over Aaron's casket to kiss his cold tender cheek goodbye was not written anywhere in our parental handbook! Especially not in the chapter dedicated to learning to let go. Neither was being thrust into the unknown world of becoming a caregiver to our twenty-two-year-old son.

In the blink of an eye, with tears streaming down my face, I sat observing my son attempt to learn the basics all over again. I anxiously waited for Steven to speak his first word. My heart wasn't prepared to hear the three words often taken for granted… "*I Love You.*" I cheered when he sat up in a chair without assistance. Each baby step of progress was a victory. I didn't dare allow my thoughts to linger on the predictions of deficits Steven might face. Instead, I focused on celebrating the reality that Steven was alive. His deficits were invisible to me. I had lost one son; I knew I wouldn't survive if I lost Steven.

Almost four years later, I admit that I was at a loss. I was angry. My heart felt shattered beyond repair. I had a plan for our sons. My plan was tucked away in a beautifully wrapped package safely secured with a big bright neatly tied bow on top. My plan consisted of watching our sons go to college, securing their dream careers. They would get married, have children, and live happily ever after. We would experience the joy of family dinners and beach vacations. Our sons would watch their Mom and Dad grow old together. Isn't that the way it's supposed to be? On August 13, 2012, my beautifully wrapped package was replaced with a package that held God's plan for our lives. I had two choices; I could attempt to return to sender, or I could dig in with both feet firmly planted and fight with every fiber of my being for Steven's second chance. I chose the latter!

After experiencing a double trauma, I was faced with learning how to let go all over again. I wanted to take Steven's pain away but couldn't. I tried to speak for him but got reprimanded. I was told Steven needed to learn how to complete tasks with one hand. I insisted that it was too soon, it would be so much easier if I did things for him. At what felt like a snail's pace Steven relearned the basics. I thrived in taking care of Steven. Keeping busy was detrimental in those early days. It was too painful to accept the reality that Aaron was gone. Without complaint, I settled into the caregiver role beautifully. I was on a mission! It never occurred to me that everything I was doing for Steven was ultimately leading me down the path of watching Steven live an independent life!

I remember the day Steven's doctor asked what he thought about driving again. I immediately thought: *Stop that*! *What a ludicrous question! What kind of doctor are you? I have already lost one son; Steven does not want or need to drive. I am taking care of him!* Steven was so gracious because he knew his mom was fragile.

Through counseling, I am learning to support Steven through each important step in his recovery, even the ones I'm not ready for. Yes, Steven got his driver's license. Each time Steven goes out the door, I wait patiently until I hear, "I made it safely, Mom." Music to my ears! To this day, Steven knows how important it is for me to hear these precious words.

Since the knock on our door, I have earned the title of being an overcomer. Against all odds I have watched my son complete

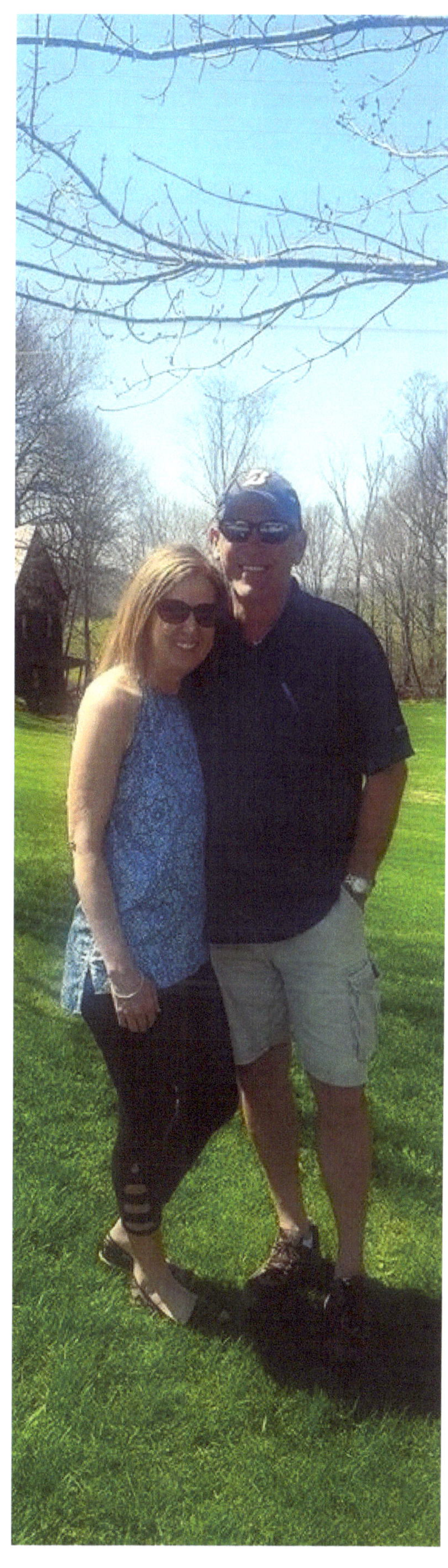

college classes, endure endless hours of grueling therapy, and bravely try every technology available to aid his recovery. When we take time to reflect on where Steven was three years ago, our focus was finding a top-notch rehab facility. The miraculous milestones Steven has achieved were never expected or voiced!

It wasn't until he was settled in at the Shepherd Center that Steven was told that Aaron didn't survive the accident. Instead of quitting, he went full speed ahead, dedicating his recovery to bring honor to Aaron's life! He has certainly gone above and beyond to do that and so much more!

There are no adequate words to describe the pain of losing one child coupled with the fear of not being able to protect your other son. I'm thankful we work together as a family, being respectful of how we each cope and adapt differently. I'm also grateful for our team of counselors. They don't pretend to know what it's like, but they dig deep to provide invaluable resources to help us learn how to let go and watch our son spread his wings and soar like a proud eagle. Will he sustain more bumps and bruises along the way? Yes, I know he will. But, I also know he will pick himself up, dust off the debris, and keep on going.

I don't know what the future holds for us. I have hopes and dreams, but this time I refuse to bundle up what I want our futures to look like in a perfectly adorned package. Instead, I will pray for our son to hold his head high as he continues down this path chosen for him. He has a happy and healthy future in front of him, helping others as he shares his story along the way! I also want Steven to witness his mother succeed at accomplishing every unsurmountable task involved in learning to let go again! Letting go doesn't mean I won't always be there for our son, it just means staying behind the scenes watching Steven independently do life. I know he will do it to the fullest, just the way it's meant to be done! When Steven's big day of changing his address arrives, and he's ready to go out our front door; for starters, I will hug him tighter and longer and with proud Momma tears, and I will say all the "*Mom*" phrases: *Be safe son, I love you, and please call when you arrive safely.*

We will get through this next chapter of life together, feeling Aaron's smile of approval every step of the way.

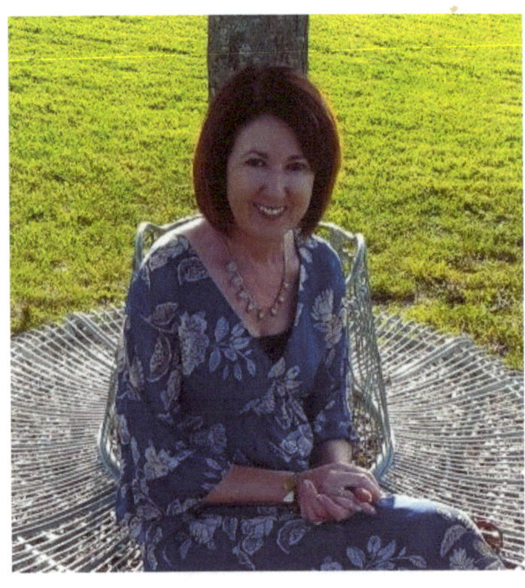

Meet Norma Myers

Norma and her husband Carlan spend much of their time supporting their son Steven as he continues on his road to recovery. Norma is an advocate for those recovering from traumatic brain injury.

Her written work has been featured on Brainline.org, a multi-media website that serves the brain injury community. Her family continues to heal.

The Ghost Within

By Dr. Katherine Kimes

There's an intimate ghost
inside me,
the spirit of my youth.
Her haunting image
lives in my reflection.
I breathe her vitality, but
her soul
no longer is mine.
Isolated
to only memories of her life,
she exists through me.
A martyr trapped
between
the solitary walls of my mind,
we share a familiar
dream.

Meet Dr. Kimes

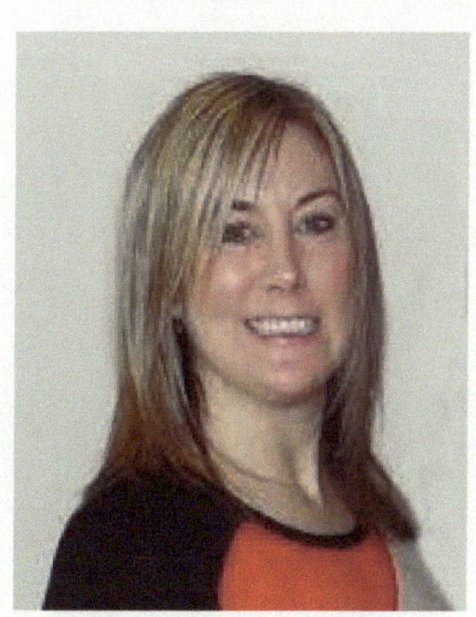

Dr. Katherine Kimes has a Master's Degree in Literary and Technical Writing from DePaul University. She also has a Master's degree in Transition Special Education with an emphasis in acquired brain injury and a Doctorate in Special Education also with a concentration in acquired brain injury. She has worked as a CSPPPD Service Coordinator and is a Certified Brain Injury Specialist.

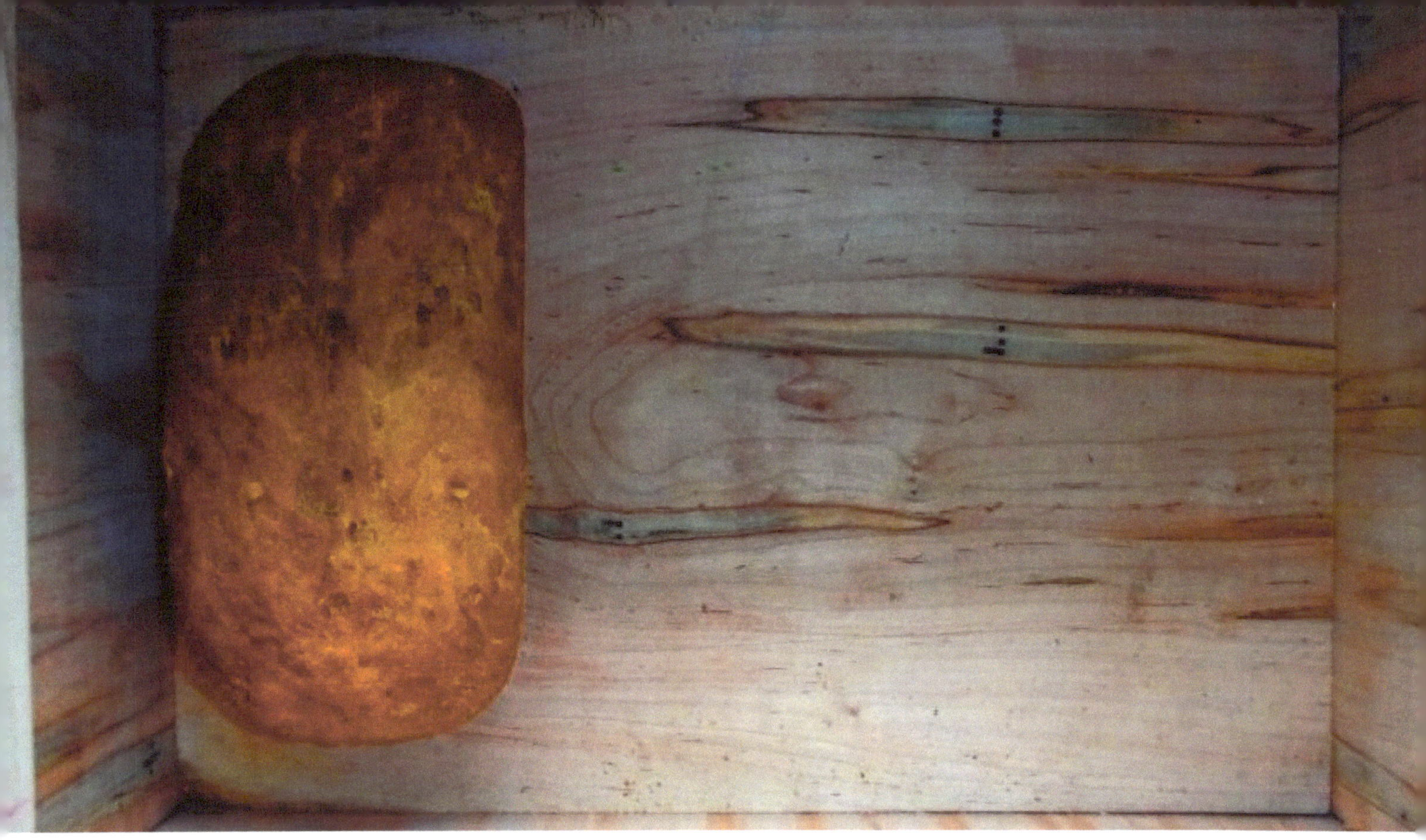

Have You Seen the Bread?

By Sarah Grant

After my husband's car accident, concussion-related challenges seemed to pop up daily. Dizziness and balance issues, constant ringing in his ears and word-finding problems started immediately. His PTSD kept us awake at night with terrifying dreams and his days were spent trying to figure out how return to work in his newly disabled body. The bills piled up and everyday life items seemed like great obstacles on our road to recovery.

As we both adjusted to our "new" life, we were also faced with the funny quirks that came along. Sometimes, he would say things that made absolutely no sense and we'd collapse into giggles – we still do this today.

> As we both adjusted to our "new" life, we were also faced with the funny quirks that came along.

Sometimes, he would say things that made me blush and if we were in public, some of those things could be inappropriate. Usually, he didn't realize that what he'd said could be hurtful or embarrassing. He was crushed if I mentioned that something may not have been the right thing to say.

It was a fine line for me to walk – ignore bad behavior and lose our friends and family or speak up and hurt his feelings. I still struggle with this one today.

During those first couple of years, we had a lot of mysteries in our house. Things would go missing – lots of things. Like forks. Spoons. So many utensils went missing that we emptied the silverware drawer during one meal. We bought new forks and spoons several times during the first five years after the accident. Since we still had children in the house, they were usually blamed for the missing utensils, missing drinking glasses, and last-roll-of-toilet-paper using. When the kids grew up and moved away and we were still scratching our heads, I realized the problem was bigger than I thought.

Through it all, we have been able to laugh and find humor in the day-to-day hurdles.

Now and then we treat ourselves to coffee "out." This isn't the kind of coffee we brew in our pot, but instead is made by someone else, exactly how we want it. My husband calls it, "Fancy coffee." During one of these coffee outings, we splurged for frozen coffees. Here in New England, there is a Dunkin' Donuts on every couple of blocks and my husband loves their Mocha Coolatta's. (He also struggled with consuming mass quantities of sugary treats soon after his accident, but that's another story.) If you're not familiar with the drink, it's made of frozen coffee, lots of cream, chocolate syrup, and then it's all blended to a slush. His always came Large and covered in whipped cream. To be clear, this isn't a diet beverage.

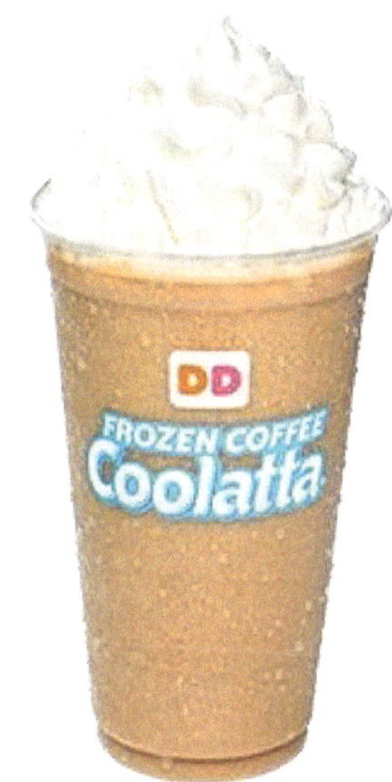

After buying our drinks that day, we took a drive out to the beach. We talked about life, our kids, the news, chores around the house, and sang along to the songs on the radio. Eventually, he reached for his Coolatta and it was empty. Still driving, he stared at me for a long time. (My drink was still mostly full.) I figured what the outcome would be, so I wasn't surprised when he finally said, "Did you drink my drink?!" This same scenario has played out over the years, with candy, French fries, and even soda's and coffee. He didn't believe my answer and we still laugh about it.

With all of the changes his brain was going through and the noise of a freight train in his ears, he was easily distracted all the time. Random things showed up where they shouldn't have. There was cheese in the cabinet. The pepper-shaker appeared in the fridge. Tennis shoes made their way to the garage as if by magic.

While making his peanut butter sandwich one day for lunch, he called me at work to say he couldn't find the bread. I'm not normally a sandwich-eater, but I was certain that we had new loaf, purchased just a couple of days prior. He was disappointed for lunch that day and it was a priority when I got home from work. Sometimes, finding things that are put away in the wrong places can be difficult. My first clue was that the toaster was on the counter. We always cleaned it after using it and tucked it into a cabinet. When I looked into the cabinet, there was the loaf of bread, ready to be eaten. Apparently, after breakfast, he put the bread away where the toaster belonged. At lunchtime, he didn't connect the relationship between the toaster being on the counter and the bread missing. He is able to realize that this happens now and will usually re-trace his steps to figure out what happened.

A couple of years ago, during a time that nothing went as planned and he was repeatedly frustrated, I started a game. An ordinary can of turkey gravy turned up in the living room, next to the television remote. It took him a couple of days to realize that it was there, but he surprised me by asking, "Did I leave this here?" I felt terrible that he thought he actually left it there, but he played the game. The next day, I found it in the bathroom. The day after that, he found it in his office, next to his phone. We didn't put it in obvious places, but we didn't hide it either. It was a way for us to make light of things. It's not his fault that he's sometimes absent-minded. If I had as much going on in my body and the noise in my ears that he does, I would be distracted too!

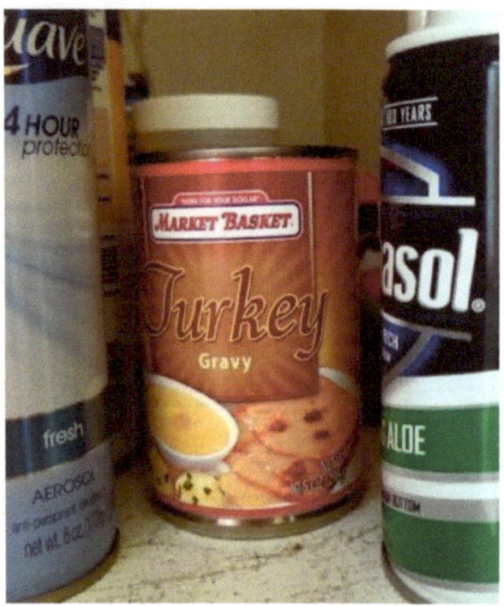

We've learned the benefits of routines, which build habits, which creates predictability. By the same token, if things are crazy busy, if we have visitors and even if we have a bad night's sleep, the "normal" is a little off-kilter and we make adjustments. Today, he frequently is able to connect the dots, but I do still find things where they don't belong. Just this morning I heard, "We must be out of bacon," followed up by, "Found it!" The package of pre-cooked bacon he has every morning for breakfast was in the freezer. Life certainly is interesting with a brain injury!

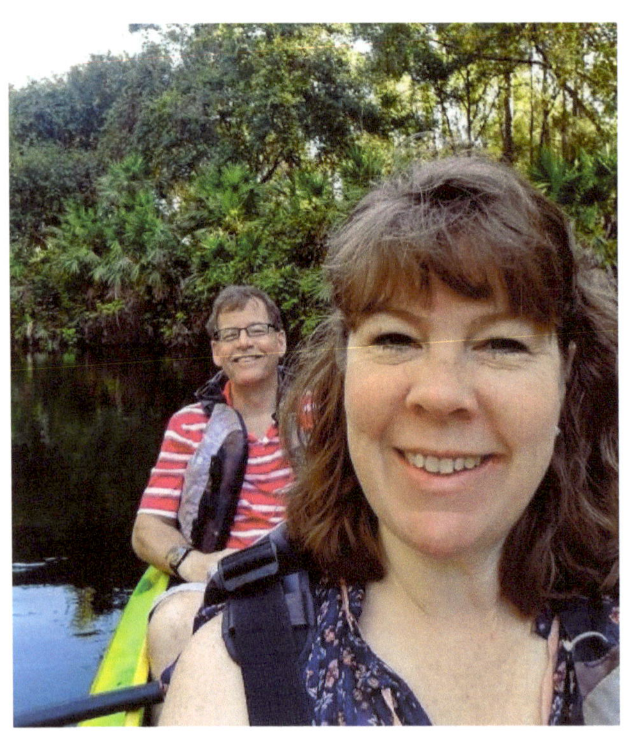

Meet Sarah Grant

Sarah lives in Salem, NH with her husband David and their two cats Belle and Boo.

She started an online Caregiver group in 2013, to help make sense of what she was experiencing, and it has since grown to almost 9,000 members around the world.

She can usually be found outdoors, enjoying life with her husband. You can learn more about Sarah's advocacy work at: www.tbicaregiversupport.com.

News & Views

This is perhaps one of the most diverse issues of HOPE Magazine to date. You've just read stories by long-term brain injury survivors and family members. This month's stories included submissions from writers both in the United States as well as Canada. Brain injury knows no borders.

We already have big plans for the October Issue of HOPE Magazine including a special section: *K9s For Warriors - Because Together We Stand.* This special section is about placing service dogs with post 9/11 veterans suffering with PTSD and TBI.

This timely article includes participants such as the National Institute of Health, the Department of Defense, the VA, the American Veteran Aid, Harvard University, Purdue University, the ASPCA.

Our goal is to serve all affected by brain injury. We would be remiss by not honoring those with brain injuries sustained in military service.

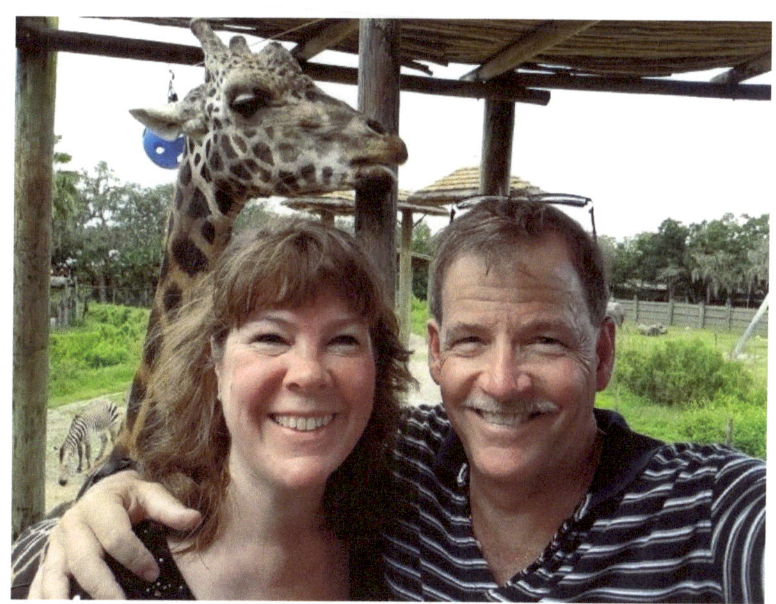

Shared before, we are always looking for courageous souls willing to share their stories with others. You can reach out to us at mystory@tbihopeandinspiration.com for more information.

To all who have supported HOPE Magazine, either by reading our magazine, or by contributing your story, we thank you. You have been a critical part of building a community that has helped and served thousands around the world.

Peace,

David & Sarah